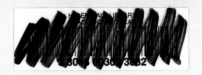

OCT   2005

EASIER

Than You

THINK

*. . . because life doesn't
have to be so hard*

BOOKS BY RICHARD CARLSON, PHD

The "Don't Sweat the Small Stuff" Series

Slowing Down to the Speed of Life (with Joseph Bailey)

Don't Worry, Make Money

You Can Be Happy No Matter What

EASIER
Than You
THINK

. . . because life doesn't have to be so hard

THE SMALL CHANGES THAT ADD UP
TO A WORLD OF DIFFERENCE

RICHARD CARLSON, PH.D.

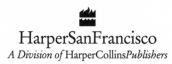

HarperSanFrancisco
A Division of HarperCollins*Publishers*

HarperCollins books may be purchased for educational, business,
or sales promotional use. For information please write: Special
Markets Department, HarperCollins Publishers, Inc., 10 East
53rd Street, New York, NY 10022.

HarperCollins Web site: http://www.harpercollins.com

HarperCollins®, 📖®, and HarperSanFrancisco™ are trademarks
of HarperCollins Publishers, Inc.

FIRST EDITION

Library of Congress Cataloging-in-Publication Data is available.

ISBN 0-06-075888-0

05 06 07 08 09 RRD(H) 10 9 8 7 6 5 4 3 2 1

I dedicate this book to my mom and dad.
You always encourage me and others to find
ways to make our lives easier.
Thank you. I love you both so much!

CONTENTS

TAKE FIVE

TURNING *on a* DIME

MY TWO BITS

INTRODUCTION
SMALL CHANGE

Most people want to change for the better—I know I do, and so do thousands of the people I've talked to. In spite of this desire to make positive changes, however, most of us are either unable or unwilling to make huge, significant changes in our already hectic lives. Let's face it, we are all too busy.

Making time for even something as simple as exercise is difficult. There's no way that I'm going to exercise for two hours a day, but I'm perfectly willing—in fact delighted—to devote twenty or thirty minutes daily in an attempt to stay fit. I'm willing to give a small amount of time because I know it makes a big difference in the quality of my day. The same can be said about so many things in life.

Take reading, for instance. How many people do you know who are going to read a hundred pages a day? My guess is, not very many. But do you suppose you could convince the average person to read ten pages a day? I'll bet you could. The truth is that most people are willing to make small, positive changes, and when they do they will be amazed by the immediate improvement in their lives.

Weeklong retreats, three-month-long diet regimens—the list of expensive and time-consuming self-improvement plans could be endless. Moreover, long-term, long-range plans for improvement come with no guarantees. That's where this book comes in. I have spent most of my adult life offering guidance to people who are looking to find happiness and harmony in their daily lives. From this work came the series of books known as *Don't Sweat the Small Stuff*. Those books are rooted in my understanding of how to thrive in the world we live in. To this day I return to them (as well as to other books, of course) when I'm feeling uptight or out of sorts and need to relax.

As with many people, my goals and priorities have grown and shifted as my life has unfolded; my sights are higher now. These past few years I have spent much of my time exploring ways to lead a more meaningful life. The book you are holding in your hands is a reflection of what I have learned in recent years.

Whereas my previous books encouraged you to take a step back so that you could gain perspective and avoid becoming upset and frustrated by life's endless details, this book encourages you to take a step forward and make an actual transformation in your life.

Transforming yourself is changing who you are on the inside, giving yourself an internal makeover. Rather than simply keeping the small stuff in life from bothering you or overwhelming you and fending off stress on a day-to-day, moment-to-moment basis—as I encouraged you to do in the *Don't Sweat* books— you can transform yourself instead into a person who isn't bothered to begin with, who doesn't even perceive the world as an inherently stressful place. Sound impossible? Well, it's really not.

We live in stressful times. Today more than ever we work longer hours, are bombarded with more

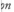

, and are anxious about the state of the this chaotic environment, we can be tempted to believe that the only way to find true peace is to escape. Most people think escape can be had in one of two ways.

One way to escape, we make the mistake of imagining, is to move away from the chaos to a more peaceful place—Hawaii or a small town, for example—or to go somewhere temporarily on vacation. The other way we escape is by "tuning out" reality through television, computers, too much work, or some other major distraction designed to take our attention away from the chaos we can't stand.

Both of these types of escape are temporary solutions that don't address the root of our stress, which, I believe, is our very response to chaos.

To be truly transformed, we need to first learn to be at peace while we're in the middle of all this confusion. Usually we are doing one of two things: either we are heading in the wrong direction or we are heading in the right direction. In other words, we are usually in either a vicious cycle or a virtuous one. When we can consciously choose to enter the eye of the storm, knowing that it may be uncomfortable at first, we can indeed learn to embrace it. By making a small change, we can alter our course, turn ourselves around, and then head off, once again, in the direction we wish to go. When we stop designing ways to avoid our problems and instead find the courage to move forward with an open mind and heart, we start to feel calm, confident, and in control.

As you begin to transform yourself into a person who doesn't experience stress and chaos in the same ways you used to, you will find that there is more love and joy in your heart. You won't have to work so hard at being loving when someone acts in an unloving way toward you. You've been transformed, so being loving comes naturally. In addition, you will have a greater appreciation for what's right with your life. You'll be transformed into a more appreciative and generous person. You will assume the innocence in others, forgive them as necessary, and want what's best for everyone—despite the fact that sometimes people do bad things. You'll see kindness and compassion as important ingredients in a successful and meaningful life. When we collectively approach the disorder of daily life in this way, we transform our world together, one person at a time.

I used to encourage people to work at becoming less reactive, and boy am I glad I did. Being less rather than more reactive is a way of being easier not only on everyone around you but on yourself as well. However, the kind of transformation I'm talking about involves less work in the long run. Once you rise above the need to be reactive, for example, you become naturally *responsive*—that's the difference. This book is about stepping forward into those places, some familiar and some less familiar, that allow you to become more peaceful and effective in a variety of ways.

As you will soon learn, this book is about far more than stress reduction. It will give you very practical, uncomplicated advice on matters that affect all aspects of your life, everything from improving your relationships with others and yourself to quieting your mind and simplifying your life, from practicing better communication skills to learning humility and discovering compassion, kindness, and the gifts of generosity. In all these aspects of life and so many more, a small change can make a huge difference.

I live in the San Francisco Bay Area, and one of my favorite things to do is to take a break from my office at lunchtime and head down to the harbor, where I can sit and watch the sailboats dart back and forth on the open water. I've always been intrigued by their beauty and precision.

A striking thing about sailboats is that the slightest movement in the rudder, or wheel, creates an enormous impact on the direction and, ultimately, the destination of the vessel. Imagine for a moment attempting to sail from San Francisco to the Hawaiian Islands—not to escape, mind you, but to discover a whole new world. It's interesting to note that if you happened to drift just a few degrees off course, you'd end up many hundreds of miles from where you wanted to be, lost in the middle of the ocean instead of gliding into a beautiful tropical bay. By making just a small, yet critical adjustment in the steering of your boat, however, you'd be able to get back on course with very little effort. In fact, making small corrections as you go is a big part of the skill involved in sailing.

Making small changes that bring great rewards to your life works, and that is what this book is all about.

In the pages that follow, I offer what I've determined to the best of my ability are the small changes that offer the most bang for the buck. The book's opening section, "A Penny for Your Thoughts," offers subtle changes you can make to your patterns of thought that can have an enormous impact on your happiness. From there we move on to "Take Five," which provides simple yet critical advice for learning how not to react out of impulse or fear but instead to respond with calm and cool to everyone from bosses to loved ones. The next section, "Turning on a Dime," details the essential changes you can make to all of your relationships that will have a remarkable impact on not only your own well-being but also the well-being of those around you. And finally, "My Two Bits" will show you once and for all that it is the little things that matter most in life.

After writing approximately twenty books and speaking to tens of thousands of people over the past fifteen years or so, I've noticed something that I find very interesting. It's something that applies to most people I meet, as well as to myself, and it's the primary reason I believe this book is so important. Making small changes is the most effective and productive way to change your life for the better. I believe you'll see right from the start that the suggestions I make are easy to set in motion yet produce the largest potential payoff. From the way you think and act to how you relate to the people you see every day and ultimately to how you interact with the world, these small changes require very little work and can fit easily into your daily schedule. If you practice them, or even just some of them, you'll begin to see changes in your life that will amaze you. You'll find that it really is the small changes, made consistently, that produce other changes that are greater than you might imagine.

Writing this book has been a tremendous learning experience for me as well as a great source of joy. I hope you will enjoy reading it as much as I have enjoyed writing it. I also hope you will consider implementing at least a few of the small changes into your life. If you do, I think you'll quickly see, not small changes, but some rather significant positive changes. It will be much smoother sailing from here on in!

A PENNY
for
YOUR THOUGHTS

———————

I.

A PENNY FOR YOUR THOUGHTS

When my daughter Kenna was a little girl, she would occasionally wake up in the morning and say to me, "Daddy, this is so great, I get another one of these!" Have you heard the expression "Out of the mouths of babes"? The excitement in my daughter's voice suggested that she was thrilled to have been given yet another day to do with what she would. Even at a tender, young age, she somehow knew that she had the choice to make each day special.

Our thoughts are the most powerful tools we have been given during this lifetime. We can use them, as Kenna did, to create joy, anticipation, excitement, fun, happiness, and peace.

Of course, we can just as easily allow our thoughts to be self-destructive weapons. We can wake up in the morning with a list of complaints as long as the front page of the newspaper. And whichever road we take—positive or negative—our choice is likely to have little if anything to do with how "good" our life really is on the "outside."

Be that as it may, our well-being depends on how we process our lives on the inside—on our thinking. What do we think? When do we think? How much significance do we give to our thinking? And most important, do we remember that we are the ones who are doing the thinking to begin with?

If you can keep in mind the reality that you control your own thoughts and nothing else, you will be in pretty good shape. Whenever negativity creeps into your mind (which it will do on a regular basis), remember two things: You are the one who is creating the negativity with your own thinking. But more important, you have the power to stop it.

Our thoughts have the power, if left to their own devices, to take us to either great heights or miserable depths. This is why it is so important to remember that we are the ones in control. We can follow our thoughts as they arise, or we can change or drop them. We alone have the choice.

I encourage you to start paying attention to the thoughts that are taking up space in your mind. Are they leading you places you want to be going? Or are they encouraging you to be unhappy, self-defeating, angry, or frustrated?

If you are having any of these feelings, or any other feeling that you wish would go away, the first place to look is not outside yourself. Instead, try to recognize what's going on inside your own mind. Once you recognize your negative thought patterns, you have the power to stop them. The change is just that simple.

Step forward and change your thoughts and you'll improve the way you feel. It's a slight shift from believing the world is going to somehow come around to your way of thinking to realizing that you are the one who must change the way you think. Bingo. What could be simpler?

Here's a case in point. Joseph was a thirty-five-year-old lab assistant who had spent most of his adult life complaining about his job and resenting everyone around him. He woke up bitter in the morning and remained that way until he went to bed. From the outside, it appeared that he had good friends, a nice apartment, and a solid job. But to hear him you would think that everything in his life was miserable.

One of his fed-up coworkers introduced Joseph to the idea that it was his own thinking, not the world, that was responsible for the endless resentment he was feeling. The coworker encouraged him to stop complaining and start paying attention to the harmful noise going on within his own mind.

Much to the relief and delight of his family, friends, and colleagues, Joseph did just that. When he was home alone, he noticed that his negative thoughts rarely let up. For the first time in his life, he was curious about his own mind. He asked himself the following questions: "Could it be possible that my own thoughts have something to do with the way I am?" And then, "Can I stop this way of thinking?" He soon learned that the answers to both were yes. And from that day forward, Joseph had much less to complain about.

A small shift in his understanding opened the door to a whole new life for Joseph, and it can for you as well. Begin paying attention to the thoughts that are going on inside your head. Whatever they happen to be, it's totally fine. There's no need to resist them. Remind yourself that your thoughts are just thoughts. Just as a check is worthless without your signature, your thoughts cannot harm you without your consent. You could be having the worst series of thoughts in the world about yourself, but if you remember that they are just thoughts and nothing else, you will be able to dismiss them, or at the very least, to give them less significance.

Once you are no longer afraid of your thinking, the transformation in your heart and mind will amaze you and every day will feel like a gift. Although this is such a small change in perception, if taken to heart, the results can truly change your life.

Let's move on. This is going to be fun.

2.

PAVING YOUR OWN WAY

Approximately 80 to 90 percent of the world's population is associated with one religion or another. Among this staggering number of people, an overwhelming majority hold the same religious beliefs as their parents and grandparents before them. I'm not making a judgment about this tendency—far from it—but rather simply noting this fascinating reality about the way in which most of us tend to make decisions. We don't usually investigate, reflect upon, or question our beliefs, opinions, and assumptions. Many of our decisions have been made for us and based as they are on our history and ideology—beliefs that have been passed from generation to generation—are absolutely predictable.

The beauty of paving your own way is that you become empowered to make independent decisions. You avoid the traps that so many of us fall into, such as unexamined bias and stubborn, habitual thinking. Most notably, you escape the trap of living someone else's life. You have the conviction of knowing that when you take a political stance, for instance, it's really yours and not simply the one you grew up with in your parents' liberal and Democratic home, or conservative and Republican one. When you think independently, you choose a career, find a relationship partner, and make other important life decisions based on your own values, wisdom, and critical thinking instead of being guided by unconscious influences. You alone decide what's important.

It's funny how we sometimes make decisions. I doubt that it's pure coincidence that my wife, Kris, and I spend the vast majority of our vacations in the same locations where our parents have spent most of theirs. And speaking of parents, if your parents went to college and pressure you to do the same, you are far more likely to move in that direction without questioning whether it's the right decision for you or not. Then there are discipline issues. If your parents were tough, there's a good chance you will be too. If your parents were lenient, so are you probably. And so it goes.

I remember a revealing conversation I had with a woman last year in the grocery store before the holidays. She was buying three hams. Making idle conversation in line, I said something like, "I guess you love ham," to which she replied, "Actually, it makes me sick to my stomach." I couldn't help but ask, "So why are you getting so much of it?" She smiled and said, "Oh, that's just what we do in our family."

Transactional analysis, a psychological theory developed by Eric Berne, claims that people are born innately healthy but develop patterns early in life based on negative or positive influences around them. These patterns are called life scripts. The best book on the subject, in my opinion, is Claude M. Steiner's *Scripts People Live*. The essential message of this book is that from an early age we fall into a role that is being played out in our family's day-to-day lives. Once this role is decided, these psychologists argue, we spend the rest of our lives playing it out. For those who fall into a negative script, the consequences can be disastrous unless a conscious decision to change is made.

Perhaps an elder member of your family said to you when you were a child, "We Smiths are military people. Your great-grandfather was in the Civil War, your grandfather was in World War I, and someday, son, you will make us proud when you fight for your country too." If you grew up hearing this, it's easy to see how difficult it would be to believe anything different. You would feel a great deal of guilt if you had failed to follow the family tradition.

What is interesting is that an adult family member doesn't necessarily have to directly state a preference, such as, "I want you to be a straight-A student," in order to have an influence on a child. When an adult continually voices his or her obvious approval of great students, scholars, and other people who have achieved academic greatness, he or she is indirectly yet no less powerfully handing down a life script.

One of the ways in which the life script takes hold is through the guilt or inadequacy a person often feels if he or she doesn't follow the script. In other words, it is far too easy to fall into patterns based on the expectations of those around us about how we are going to think and act. The small change of paving your own way is accomplished when you realize that you are being guided instead of creating your own destiny. This small change will alter your life in a very big way.

Living your life based on your own individual dreams and desires is critical for happiness. Learning to think and act, not out of habit, but with your own creative and independent ideas is powerfully transformative. Here are two simple ways to break free:

1. Resist the urge to make decisions quickly. Whenever we react, we almost always speak out of habit. For example, if someone says to me, "Richard, where would you like to go on vacation?" my immediate answer is likely to be, "The ocean." Why? That's where we usually go. And that's where we always went when I was growing up. Is this a bad thing? No, but if I want to be open to new experiences, it would be helpful to stop and think for a moment about where I truly would like to go. Perhaps I'd still choose the

ocean, but without actually stopping and thinking, I'll never know.

2. Gather opinions from people who have different points of view and have had different experiences. When we ask for advice or solicit feedback, we are almost always drawn to those who already agree with our point of view. All this kind of advice does, however, is reinforce your preexisting decision. Hearing differing opinions and perspectives will help you break out of the rut of rote thinking. You can end up agreeing, but your opinion will be your own.

3.

BE THERE FOR YOURSELF

Cathy was nice to just about everyone except one person—herself. She was thoughtful, patient, kind, and caring. She would surprise friends with loving cards, call those she cared about just to say hi, and send gifts to friends and family on special occasions. She rarely, however, did anything nice for herself. Not only that, she would regularly berate herself for anything she perceived that she did wrong and talk to herself in negative ways. In short, she treated herself as she would treat someone she really didn't like, and these habits had translated into low self-confidence.

As the years went by, Cathy slowly became tired

and a bit resentful. The reality of how she treated herself finally caught up with her, and she no longer had the love and the energy it took to please everyone.

When I first met Cathy, however, she was so positive to both herself and those around her that I was shocked when she told me about her transformation. A close friend had introduced Cathy to a wonderful therapist who shared with her one of the most important "small change" secrets in the universe: you can give to others only what you yourself have to give. And one of the best ways to have more love to give is to first give that love to yourself.

It's sad, but of all the people in our lives, perhaps the person most of us are the hardest on, pay the least attention to, and shower the least amount of love upon is ourselves.

When we are kind, and take time for ourselves, we have something left over for other people. If we don't love ourselves, we can't offer much in the way of love to others.

You can become kinder to yourself in two ways. First, avoid sabotaging yourself with negativity and self-loathing by indulging in self-deprecating and self-defeating statements. Thoughts such as "I can't do it" and "I haven't been a very good friend (partner, parent, child, etc.)" also take up an awful lot of band-width on many people's "inner airwaves." When you start paying attention on a regular basis to what you are thinking, you may be shocked at how often you think negatively about yourself.

When you catch yourself thinking negatively, drop the thought from your mind and then pat yourself on the back. All of us have innate self-esteem that kicks in as soon as we stop being hard on ourselves. Ask yourself the question, "Am I being as kind to myself as I would be to a good friend?" If the answer is no, it's time to ask, "Why?" and to change your priorities.

The second way to become kinder to yourself is to reserve time in your day or week just for you. The spe-cific form of the kindness isn't as important as the kindness itself. Whether it's time spent in quiet re-flection, reading, prayer or meditation, regular exer-cise, making a trip to your favorite bookstore, or taking a hot bubble bath, it's important that you find time to do nice things just for yourself. Acknowledge that you deserve special treatment and that you have earned the kindness that you undoubtedly try so hard to give to others.

Far from being selfish, your loving-kindness toward yourself will trigger your natural instinct to want to give that love back to others.

When Cathy started taking time for herself—taking walks, reading books, getting an occasional massage, and spending time with friends—she became happier, and her love for others returned in abundance.

Remember, what goes around comes around. When it comes to kindness, it all starts with you. This easy change is well worth the effort.

4.

YOUR LIFE CAN CHANGE AT
THE DROP OF A HAT

Sudden change is often a difficult subject to talk about in front of a group because a certain percentage of the audience believes I'm being a little pessimistic. I can assure you, I'm not.

It's critical that we realize that at any moment our lives can change. Realistically, there will come a time when our everyday life will suddenly be altered. We just don't know when it will be.

Many of us will get that dreaded phone call, giving us some piece of bad news. Maybe you'll hear from your doctor that something is wrong with you. Or maybe you will unexpectedly lose your job.

Change also goes both ways. Your life can be altered for the better in an instant. When you least expect it, you might meet a new friend, fall madly in love, come up with a brilliant idea, or discover a new career direction. You just never know, and this is one of the reasons why life is so exciting and mysterious.

Far too many of us dread the idea of change. We like things just the way they are. However, whether we like it or not, things are going to change. Living life with the awareness that things are going to change helps prepare you for the unavoidable. Rather than being shocked or thrown off when a change comes, you can react with an unruffled sense of acceptance.

I'll never forget the time I was sitting with my colleague Paul when he received an unexpected call from his lawyer informing him that he was going to lose his house to foreclosure. He was a little behind in his payments, had recently lost his job, and was without a doubt down on his luck. Amazingly, it seemed as though I felt worse about the foreclosure than he did. His acceptance of the news and the situation was something to behold. He was calm and collected and went about his business as usual.

After I was certain that his reaction was for real and that he was not putting up a false front for my sake, I asked him how he was managing to remain so calm. He told me he had learned long ago that one of the most important lessons in life is that eventually everything changes. "The only question," he said, "is when." He went on to say that the "when" in his case was now. Even with crisis bearing down on him, he was able to remind me of this life lesson.

Every day each of us is subjected to situations in which the underlying issue is the simple fact that life is changing. Fortunately, the issue isn't usually as significant as losing our home or someone we love. If we can remember that change is a constant, it will help us tackle all the changes, both big and small, that come our way.

It is important to remember that change is not only inevitable but also something that we can prepare for. I know that might sound weird, but stay with me. Here are some simple ways to prepare. Go through your closets and give away all those things you no longer need and have held on to for too long.

Notice that, as you let go of these items, even if you're a little uncomfortable at first, everything is okay. In fact, cleaning out the closet feels pretty good. You're learning that, although change can seem difficult and unwanted, it can also lead to pleasant surprises.

Now try an interpersonal experiment. Think of someone you used to be close to but with whom your relationship faltered over time. Perhaps you had several small disputes over the years, and now the two of you rarely if ever speak. Consider making a change and summoning the courage to initiate communication. Give that person a call or write her a letter. Break the ice. If you do this, and the intention is genuine, you will have changed the energy between the two of you from negative to positive. You may have dreaded making that phone call or putting pen to paper, but often just making the effort results in a positive change.

Change happens. Our job is to remember that it is a constant and that how we react to it often helps determine whether it is positive or negative.

Knowing that life can and does change at the drop of a hat is a powerful tool. With this knowledge, you can participate in making changes in your life rather than simply waiting for life to happen. And when life does spring surprises on you, this awareness allows you to respond to what comes at you more flexibly and with an open heart.

5.

THE MOST BASIC
CHOICE OF ALL

As I was reflecting on the small changes each of us can make in our lives, the one that stood out was the most basic of all. It's the decision we make every single day when we wake up about how to approach the day. Are we going to feel sorry for ourselves, or are we going to take responsibility for our own happiness? Are we going to look for what's wrong and find it? Or are we going to look for what's right and find that instead? Will we see the problems or the opportunities? Will we be part of the problem or part of the solution? Will we be judgmental about life or accepting?

All these questions, and so many more like them, can be bundled up into one package called attitude. And attitude can be summed up in one word— choice. Choosing to change our attitude may seem like a small change, but it can't happen unless we recognize that it's all up to us. Do we realize that we have the choice to make our day joyful, adventuresome, exciting, and full of magic? Or do we demand that life be a certain way, and if it doesn't meet our expectations we whine and complain?

My dear friend John Welshons, author of one of the most profound books I've ever read, *Awakening from Grief,* told me the following story, shared with him originally by an old friend who didn't know who the original author was. Do pay close attention to the conscious choices the author makes in this story and think about how easily he or she could have made other choices.

I woke up early today excited about all I get to do before the clock strikes midnight. I have responsibilities to fulfill today. My job is to choose what kind of day I'm going to have. I can complain because the weather is rainy, or I can be thankful that the grass is getting watered for free.

Today I can feel sad that I don't have more money, or be glad that my finances encourage me to plan my purchases wisely and to guide me away from waste. Today I can grumble about my health, or I can rejoice that I am alive. Today I can lament over all my parents didn't give me when I was a child, or I can be grateful that they allowed me to be born.

Today I can cry because roses have thorns, or I can celebrate that thorns have roses. Today I can whine because I have a job, or I can *shout* for joy because I have a job to do! Today I can complain because I have to go to school, or I can eagerly open my mind and fill it with new tidbits of knowledge. Today I can murmur dejectedly because I have to do housework, or I can feel honored because the Lord has provided shelter for my mind and body and soul. Today stretches ahead of me waiting to be shaped, and here I am the sculptor who gets to do the shaping. What today will be like is up to me. I get to choose what kind of day I will have. So have a great day—unless you have other plans.

When you get right down to it, we either believe we are the choice maker or we don't. When you see the rampant unhappiness and victimization in our culture, it's clear that most people don't see that we do have this choice. At the same time, when you take a step back and think about it, it's pretty obvious. If we aren't the choice maker, who is? If we don't decide what kind of a day we're going to have, who does?

That's why this subtle shift in thinking is one of the more significant changes we will ever make. For me, consciously choosing a better attitude has made a world of difference, and I know it can for you as well. Think about the implications. You can choose to complain about your teenager, or you can thank God that you have a teenager to love. Kids can be difficult, but you wouldn't trade yours for the world. Why choose the path of complaint over the path of gratitude?

Even with mundane things the same principle applies. When I remind myself that I'm the choice maker, it puts everything into perspective. I can complain that I'm spending too much time driving kids around in my car. Or I can marvel at how lucky I am to be among the privileged people on this earth who own a car.

You can make an articulate argument for either side—being grateful or being overextended. One will lead you toward satisfaction, and the other toward guaranteed and sustained grief. And the beautiful part is that you get to make the choice.

EASIER THAN YOU THINK

6.

REMEMBER THE POWER OF HOPE

Hope is one of the most powerful forces in our lives. It keeps us happy instead of depressed, looking toward the future instead of the past, and knowing there's always a chance that life can be better than it is right now regardless of our circumstances. Hope keeps the human spirit alive. It gives us reason to go on even when times are tough. It keeps us enthused, inspired, and optimistic. It also gives us reason to give others another chance even when they have done something wrong or when it seems they might not "deserve" it.

A friend of mine shared with me the following quote from Archbishop Desmond Tutu, who worked all his life to change the system of apartheid in South Africa. It has become one of my favorites, and I keep a copy of it in several locations—in my home, in my office, and in my car. I read it almost every day. Here's what Archbishop Tutu said:

> There is no situation that is not transformable. There is no person who is hopeless. There is no set of circumstances that cannot be turned about by ordinary human beings and their natural capacity for love of the deepest sort.

Perhaps the most remarkable aspect of hope is that it's entirely internal. Many prisoners who have experienced unimaginable fear have maintained the hope that someday they would somehow get out of prison. Because of that hope, they were somehow able to survive. Parents who have experienced any nightmare involving the health or well-being of a child have survived the ordeal largely because of their hope that their child would someday be okay.

In everything from these extremely painful situations down to everyday situations, hope soothes the soul. For instance, we might be under consideration for a promotion at work. We're excited, anxious, and nervous, all at the same time. What gets us through the roller-coaster ride of emotions in one piece is hope. We hope we will get the job. The hope is the positive energy that keeps us motivated and enthused while we wait. And if we don't get the job, it's hope once again that tells us we might have a shot next time. Hope is that invisible force that makes all things possible.

I heard a tragic yet inspiring story about a little boy in Sudan, Africa, whose village had been taken over by a group of rebels. They had killed almost every person in the village, including the little boy's parents and other family members. Somehow the little boy survived under a pile of rubble, pretending to be dead.

With very little food or water, the little boy traveled by foot for hundreds of miles because he was once told by his parents that his village had a sister village on the mouth of the river and that he should escape to this village in case of emergency. All he had was hope and his own strength. It took weeks of walking and all the hope and strength he could muster, but he made it. His hope carried him through, and the new village gave the young boy a new place to call home.

In the end, whether we're talking about something really huge or something relatively minor, as Archbishop Tutu maintains and as this little boy surely believed, "there is always hope, and this will be solved." Because hope is created in our own hearts and minds, we are in control of it and can create more of it if we choose to.

As an experiment, I want you to think about something in your life that you are worrying about. Now, instead of sending the same old worried energy toward those thoughts, send some hopeful energy toward them instead. For example, suppose your current worry has to do with a conflict with a family member. Let's say that every time you get together with your aunt Mary, the two of you argue and you end up getting upset.

This time, however, it's going to be different. You have a family reunion coming up, and you're both going to be there. Instead of worrying, as you normally do, about what's going to happen between you and aunt Mary, practice sending positive thoughts and energy in her direction instead. Close your eyes and see yourself with Mary, and see the two of you getting along just beautifully. No matter what she says or does, your response will be loving.

Think, once again, about Desmond Tutu's words: "There is no set of circumstances that cannot be turned about by ordinary human beings and their natural capacity for love of the deepest sort."

This means that even if your aunt isn't perfect, or if she drinks too much, or if she says something out of line, or if she falls into an old habit, it doesn't matter. You don't need Mary to change, because you hold all the cards you need—you have the capacity to change things by virtue of the love within your heart. Any and all bitterness, resentment, jealousy, or just difficult family dynamics will fade away as a direct result of the love that grows within you. All you have to do is maintain the hope that things will be better this time. I'd be willing to bet that if you hold this thought in your mind, things will indeed be better.

You have nothing to worry about. Your hope will be contagious and spread to everyone you touch. That's the best part of all of this. None of us has to worry about changing other people. All of that will take care of itself if we foster the love and hope within ourselves.

As an added experiment, try spending a minute or two minutes every day consciously hoping for something positive in your life. Hope not for something material, such as a new car or a promotion, but for something spiritual, such as having more peace of mind or getting along better with your neighbors and those in your family. By spending just a few minutes a day with this type of positive energy, you'll be creating a positive environment for a happier life. Though engaged in a small action, you'll be part of a very large solution.

7.

"I WON'T GO THERE"

There are times when it's important to take yourself places with your mind, and there are other times when you are better off telling yourself, "I won't go there." These four simple words can change your life. This simple phrase has profound results.

Two of our dearest friends and neighbors, Chris and Mark, experienced every parent's worst nightmare in the summer of 2002. The phone rang in the middle of the night, and they were told that their youngest son, Mario, who was eighteen, had been involved in a horrible automobile accident. He had hit a telephone pole head on while traveling at a high speed. When he arrived at the hospital, he was pronounced dead but then was miraculously brought back to life. Mario was on life support for days, and there were many people, including several members of the hospital staff, who believed he would never make it. Well, Mario did make it, but the recovery has been slow and painful.

In the years since the accident there have been an unlimited number of opportunities for Chris and Mark to feel sorry for themselves, to convince themselves that life is too hard, or to just give up. Every day Mario's family could dwell on any of dozens of frightening and unanswerable questions such as "What is Mario going to do five years from now?" or "How are we going to afford this long-term?"

Recently I was outside watering my plants when I got to talking with Mario's dad. During the course of our conversation, I asked Mark what has enabled him to keep so strong and wise during this entire ordeal. Without pause, he said with a smile, "Four simple words: 'I won't go there.' Truthfully, that's our secret. We simply don't allow ourselves to go down that path of worry and dread. Since the situation is tough enough, allowing our minds to take us to even more difficult scenarios would make life almost unbearable."

Their strategy has paid off substantially. A year and a half later, Mario is learning to communicate and to use his body again, and most important of all, his spirits are high. Every time I see him he's happy to be alive. In fact, he may be the happiest person I know.

Chris and Mark are not pretending that their situation is easy, nor are they denying that it's demanding. What they have done instead is to minimize their pain and suffering by refusing to let their minds take them into a state of unending worry and dread. Many of us have legitimate concerns and experience real pain, but we still don't have to dwell on worst-case scenarios. We can all take Mark's advice and "not go there."

No matter what your situation is, making this small change will help you focus better on what is right in front of you and will ultimately lead you to a happier, more productive life.

8.

WATCH YOUR THOUGHTS

This is one of the most entertaining strategies in this entire book. The idea of watching your thoughts might sound odd at first, but you will soon see that this is a very accurate description of a very useful tool. And once you get the hang of watching your thoughts, it will become one of the most powerful tools available to you.

This technique has been around for as long as people have been meditating. Watching your thoughts is a small change that offers you the amazing opportunity to stop the wheels from turning every second and gain critical perspective. The payoff will change your life for good. Here's how it works.

The technique itself is not complicated, and don't let anyone convince you otherwise. Imagine going to a theater and watching a movie. You can be completely immersed in the movie and yet a part of you is totally detached. If you're watching the latest horror movie about giant sea monsters, you obviously don't feel compelled to bring scuba tanks and underwater guns to the theater. Why? Because you are detached enough to know the movie is just a movie.

When you start watching your own thoughts as you would a movie, this same detachment allows you to witness the many thoughts that occur in your brain, but without being overcome by these thoughts. What you come to realize is that you have an infinite number of thoughts each day, and many vie for your attention simultaneously. It's as if one is yelling out to you, "Pay attention to me," while another is saying, "No, pay attention to me." This realization, like the scary movie, can be frightening. The good news, however, is that, just like the movie, these are only thoughts. And as you watch thought after thought enter your mind, you realize that you can quiet the inner noise they make. This is where the importance of detachment comes in.

Over time, and with a little practice, you can get to the point where you treat your own thoughts much like the movie you watch at the theater. You can be totally responsive to them, yet detached enough to keep your bearings and not allow your thoughts to drive you nuts.

Let me give you an everyday and personal example of how watching your thoughts works. A few weeks ago, two very dear friends of mine separately asked me to do them a favor on the same day. At first I welcomed the chance to help out. It's rare that either of these friends asks me to do anything for them, and both are always there for me. The problem was that both favors were being "called in" at the exact same time! There was no way around it. If I was to help one friend, I would have to let the other friend down.

Obviously this wasn't a life-or-death dilemma, but you can probably imagine what my mind started to do. My thoughts began going in about six different directions, and each thought seemed perfectly logical as it called out to me, "This is why you should do it this way." Then, not a tenth of a second later, another thought would jump in and say, "But, Richard, you can't possibly not be there for John; he's never once not been there for you." When I imagined saying no to both requests, a few self-loathing thoughts sneaked into the mix, such as "How can you possibly be so selfish?"

Fortunately, about five minutes into this potentially endless agony, I remembered the technique of watching my thoughts. Instead of engaging my thoughts any further, I simply started to observe them. It was as if I stepped back and removed myself from the picture. I did nothing else but watch. Within a few minutes my thoughts began to slow down. My mind quieted, and the situation seemed less like an emergency.

Shortly thereafter, I knew it would all work out just fine. I trusted that I would make the right decision, which, as it turned out, I did. I was able to be with one friend and, explaining the situation, had a heart-to-heart phone conversation with the other.

Every day we must deal with hundreds of competing thoughts. The small change we can make is to stop trying to engage every thought that pops into our mind and stop trying to figure out every drama in our mind. Instead, we can simply step back and watch the show. It's really just like watching that movie on the screen.

You can go as far as you want to with this technique. It can be a tool you use on occasion to deal with the stress that builds up during the day. Or you can make it an integral part of your everyday life.

The next time you become agitated, worried, harried, or simply unable to focus, step back and watch your thoughts. The results will amaze you. With just this subtle shift, you can move from stress and uncertainty to resolution, calm, and joy.

9.

THE GRASS IS AS GREEN
AS IT NEEDS TO BE

Recently I attended a fund-raising event. Despite the upbeat purpose of the event and the large number of generous attendees, I was amazed at how many people there were focused not on what their life *is*, but on what it *isn't*. It was a shock to hear so many bighearted and charitable folks talk about what's missing.

If you listen carefully, too many of our conversations seem to inexorably shift focus to what's wrong with life, or to how life is not living up to our expectation about how it's supposed to be. Whether the conversation has to do with our bodies not being the right size, or not having enough money, the right job, the right house, or the right neighbors, this social habit manifests in dozens of ways.

Often dissatisfaction shows up in how we feel about other people. "They," we'll say, are "weird" or "strange" or "don't cut it." At the fund-raising event, several people discussed with me their dissatisfaction with their daughters' or sons' choice of boyfriend or girlfriend, husband or wife. Others were unhappy with their own spouse. It seemed like very few people were "good enough." One person who was obviously very generous was criticizing himself for not giving as much money this year as he had in previous years!

Many of those at this event complained bitterly about taxes, the liberals or the conservatives, or the "evil" politicians. Mostly, however, people talked about how life would be better if certain conditions were met, such as if the weather were better, or the economy or stock market were more robust. Some wished there was less greed in the world, or nicer people, and so forth.

I'm not passing judgment, only making an observation. I've done this kind of thing many times myself.

You name it, and I've probably complained about it. What I've learned, however, is that what happens 100 percent of the time when I complain about life is that my spirits are lowered. Now when I catch myself in the act of complaining, I'm usually able to realize that I'm not getting anywhere as a result.

I'm sure many of you are familiar with this saying: the grass is always greener on the other side of the fence. For years I've referred to this type of thinking as the "if-only-then trap." It's a trap because if you base your happiness on things being different than they are currently, you've set yourself up for constant disappointment. A more accurate saying would be: the grass is exactly the same color on the other side of the fence.

A man once said to me, as if he were proud of it, "I'll never be happy as long as my daughter is married to that bum." I wasn't quite sure what to say because, although I didn't know his daughter and her husband very well, they sure appeared to be happy together. By the looks of things, this man was destined for a life of self-imposed misery.

I don't think any of us set out to be miserable. In

fact, I'm quite certain we don't. Yet whenever we demand that life be different than it is right now, we're setting our own trap. I know I've done this to myself on many occasions. Perhaps you have too.

Perceiving the grass as greener on the other side of the fence is not the same as having preferences, or working hard to improve certain aspects of our lives, or changing the things we wish to change. All of these choices make perfect sense. But to base our happiness on things we cannot control and to demand that life accommodate our preferences—well, that is a different story.

If we can accept the fact that the grass is as green as it needs to be and that it's possible for us to be happy right now, then our lives will be easier. Focusing on what is wrong as opposed to what is right leads to a never-ending cycle of frustration. There are things we simply cannot change or control no matter how much we would like to. If we let these things take over, we are choosing to make ourselves unhappy.

There is a substantial reward for appreciating your day-to-day life just the way it is. Your level of dissatisfaction will lessen proportionally as you stop thinking that the grass is greener just over the fence. If you practice being happy with the life you have today, right now, you will be amazed by what happens. You'll get the satisfaction and contentment you've been postponing for so long.

TAKE FIVE

IO.

TAKE FIVE

One of the things that becomes more apparent over the years is the fact that we have very little control over what happens around us. As our kids grow up, we lose control over their decisions. Most of the time we don't have a say in what our colleagues do. The economy has booms and busts. The weather can ruin plans we have had for months. Just by living our everyday lives, we are affected by so many things—some good, some not so good—that we have no control over. The only solution is to let go.

The best we can do is what I like to call "take five." Another way of saying this is that we need to create the emotional space within ourselves to be able to respond to life rather than just react to it. By immediately reacting to people and events that we have no control over, we are fighting a battle we are going to lose. But by taking five, standing back and getting perspective, we gain an understanding of the situation at hand and realize the best way to move forward.

This simple distinction can be the difference between a peaceful existence and one marked by inner turmoil, between harmony and strife, between knowing the best course of action and flailing helplessly in the wind.

Consider the following story. Dave and Rebecca both worked in the marketing department of a major food company and shared the same boss. The boss had one major flaw. Robert was described by many who knew him as "the worst listener in the entire world." I can partially vouch for the validity of this claim, since I've met a number of other people who reported to him and met him myself on one occasion. Immediately, I could see what both Dave and Rebecca were saying. When you spoke to Robert, it was as if he were on a different planet. Whether or not he was this way intentionally, it was clear he was ignoring you.

But the Roberts of the world will always exist. What I want to do here is compare Dave's and Rebecca's reactions when put in the position of having to work for Robert, which neither of them wanted to be doing.

Dave hated every minute of his job and let you know about it every chance he got. When he wasn't working side by side with Robert, he might as well have been. Dave thought about Robert constantly. He kept track of the number of times he felt ignored by Robert and then would tell others about it later that day, including his wife after he got home.

When Dave ran into someone he considered a good listener, he would immediately compare that person to Robert. He told himself and those around him that he would never be happy as long as he had to work for that jerk. He allowed Robert to interfere not only with his work but with every other aspect of his life as well. Clearly he took Robert's poor listening skills very personally.

Rebecca dealt with the situation very differently. Although she disliked Robert and the fact that she had to work for someone who was such an awful listener, she recognized that it was really Robert's problem, not hers. She didn't take his poor listening skills personally because she could clearly see that Robert didn't listen to anyone—not her, not his other employees, not his own boss, not even his own family, who had stopped by the workplace a few times over the past year.

Another major difference between Rebecca and Dave was that the only time I heard Rebecca mention Robert's name was when I asked her about him. When I brought this to her attention, she laughed out loud! She said, "You must be kidding. I get enough of him at work. There's no way I'm going to take him with me every time I get to leave this place."

Because Rebecca didn't think about Robert when she wasn't at work and didn't commiserate with others about him, she could differentiate her dealings with her boss from the rest of her job. To that end, she claimed that she loved her job, at least most of it. "In fact," she said, "I even like Robert. You just have to see him as innocent and realize that he's not ignoring you on purpose. He doesn't really mean any harm."

If we go through life as reactive people like Dave, we're going to have an extremely difficult time. After all, the world just keeps on happening, and we have so little control over the events in it. There are always going to be people doing things we don't like and things happening that we wish were different.

The truth is that the only aspect of life you have any control over is your own reaction to the events taking place. If you can learn to become more responsive to life and not take it all personally, as Rebecca has learned to do with Robert, your life is going to be much smoother and a lot easier.

"Taking five" is about learning to choose between jumping up and down in protest, reacting to life as if everything taking place is about you, and taking a moment, gathering yourself, and responding with a clear understanding of what you can control.

"Taking five" involves nothing more than stepping back. We don't control much of what happens around us, but we do control how we respond to it. Knowing that we have this choice—not some of the time but all of the time—brings with it a tremendous feeling of peace and security.

II.

TAKE A VACATION EVERY DAY

Suppose you have twenty things to do during the course of a day. Further, suppose that nineteen of those things go well. The question is, which of the twenty things do most of us tend to focus on when we get home at night? Which do we talk about with those we love?

The answer, of course, is that most of us tend to focus on the one or two things that went wrong instead of the overwhelming number of things that went right. Why? Because we've become accustomed to spending our time and mental energy zeroing in on all that's wrong and all that needs to be done.

It's time to create a new habit. Even if the good outweighs the bad, we spend the majority of our energy focusing on what went wrong. That's why it is time to take ourselves on what I call mini-vacations.

We don't have to be on a cruise or in a cabin in the woods to relax and enjoy ourselves. Instead, we can easily set aside short periods of time each day and bring fun and balance back into our lives. Not to escape, as I mentioned in the introduction to this book, but to be kind to ourselves and take time out to remember that life is often good.

A friend of mine works very long hours. Every morning before work, he listens to loud classical music on his stereo for at least a half-hour while he gets ready for his day. He loves it and considers this his time. It brings him great satisfaction. You may love music too, but your choice may be rock and roll. Fantastic. Another friend loves to take snowshoe walks in the cold of winter when he can. While some are complaining about the weather, he considers the icy cold a true blessing!

Whatever you do on your mini-vacation, if it gives you a break during your day, it's perfect for you. It is your special time, and, if possible, make it non-negotiable. In other words, don't let other priorities interfere unless they are true emergencies.

Mini-vacations can also involve other people. You might want to meet friends for coffee or lunch or take a short walk early in the morning. Whether it's surfing the Internet, going for a run, playing a board game with friends, watching the sunrise, taking the dog for a walk, meditating, sitting down to a cup of tea, or cooking, doing anything that relaxes you is like taking a mini-vacation. It's a reset button that helps you de-stress.

When we take mini-vacations every day, life isn't nearly as overwhelming. We have something to look forward to that is a perfect antidote to our results-obsessed lives.

This is a very small change in terms of minutes expended, yet the energy, enthusiasm, and vitality it produces will astound you.

12.

NOTICE WHAT GETS YOU

People get so stressed out by the silliest things. A friend of mine gets bent out of shape when her fork is too small. But I can't laugh at her. I get irritated when my voice-mail box fills up faster than I can empty it. Then again, I know people who are bugged by the way people park their cars on the street, the way grocery stores stock food items, and the way advertisements try to get our attention. The list goes on and on and on.

One of the most powerful observations I've ever made about stress is this: obsessing over what stresses us out can cause more stress than what originally made us stressed to begin with. I know that's a mouthful, but it is true. And once you see the wisdom in this statement, your life will never be the same. It goes to the heart of what really causes stress.

Think about all the things that bother you on a day-to-day, moment-to-moment basis. For most of us the bothersome things are virtually unlimited. In other words, almost anything might stress us out—anything from opinionated or loud people to bad drivers to the way people dress to people who wave their hands around when they speak. Or full voice-mail boxes or small forks.

If you start paying attention to the events, statements, and behaviors that get to you, you'll soon realize that it is not these specific things that cause you stress but rather the way you react to them. So rather than react as you normally do—getting frustrated, angry, and stressed out—simply take note of where you get bothered and when exactly you feel like you are dying to react.

Become an observer of your own reactions. At first you may not even be aware that you have been thrown off course until many hours after the fact. Then all of a sudden you'll say to yourself something like "Wow,

I really lost it" or "Boy, was I caught up." It's okay if it takes you a little time to get to this point. What's important is that you are able to see what happened and to know that the stress was caused not by the external event itself but by your own mind being stuck on it.

In time, the gap between being upset and noticing what made you upset will get smaller and smaller. Most of our knee-jerk reactions are due to a lack of awareness. It's not the object of my frustration—the voice-mail box—but the fact that I'm caught up in my thinking about it that makes me upset. Therefore, the act of being aware that I'm caught up in my thinking is a powerful antidote to a huge percentage of my stress. Noticing the source of my stress for what it is—something not real—seems to send a signal to my brain that says, "Don't worry about it."

The first and most important step in eliminating a great deal of stress from your life is simply becoming aware of what stresses you out. You might think it's a pretty small change to pay attention to what gets you. In fact it is, but you'll soon see that it produces some pretty staggering results. And once you know what is making you stressed, you may just find it funny.

13.

RECOGNIZE WHEN
YOU'RE FIGHTING REALITY

After a lecture in Chicago one evening, I was speaking to a forty-seven-year-old man from the audience who had a twenty-year-old son. This nice man, named William, was telling me how disappointed he was that his son had decided not to attend college. He said that it was "his dream" that his son not make the same mistake he had.

William went on to say that he knew not going to college was the worst decision he had ever made and that he was certain his son would never recover if he made the same mistake. I could see in this man's eyes that he believed what he was saying, that his pain was real, and that it was severe.

The fact of the matter was that William's son wasn't going to college. It was obvious that nothing this father could do or say was changing that fact. The problem was that William was fighting against certainty.

Learning to recognize when we are arguing with, or struggling against, reality may be one of the smallest shifts you can make in your attitude. But it may also yield one of the most significant insights. Very simply, recognizing when you're fighting reality spells the difference between guaranteed misery and a life filled with peace and contentment.

Think about what happens whenever any of us argue with reality, when we resist what is. We might dwell on how much we hate the fact that the new neighbor has moved in down the street, or that the liberals or the conservatives are in charge of Congress (as the case may be). The problem is that the neighbor has moved in down the street, and the liberals or the conservatives are in charge, just as William's son has decided not to attend college. In any of these cases, it's

EASIER THAN YOU THINK

eye-opening to ask the question: how is resisting concrete reality going to help? Or to put it even more bluntly, is there any chance whatsoever that fighting reality is going to make you feel better? The answer is—and will always be—no.

You can hate the truth, and you can talk about it and resist it until you're blue in the face. You can complain and look for sympathy, stomp your feet, feel like a victim, and spend the rest of your life feeling sad, depressed, angry, and resentful. But none of this is going to change anything.

Being aware of the difference between what we can control and what we can't is critical for day-to-day happiness. There is no point in banging our heads against a wall. Once we understand what we can't do, we can then make the most important decisions about what we will do. Instead of fighting with his son, for instance, William could have simply shared his concerns and worked with him to ensure that the decision to skip college did not damage his future.

It's a subtle shift in your thinking to be able to recognize when you're fighting reality, and the fact is that most of us do it a great deal of the time. But if you can make that slight change in your awareness, you will save yourself a great deal of agony and empower yourself and your decisions like never before.

14.

FOCUS ON THE BLESSINGS

As I've traveled around the country speaking to different audiences about not sweating the small stuff, I've noticed that many people tend to focus so much on what's wrong with their lives—their jobs, their relationships, and other circumstances—that they fail to notice what's going right.

It is often necessary to focus on what's wrong in order to make things better. But ask yourself these questions: Are you dwelling on what's wrong because you're genuinely trying to improve things? Or are you focused on all that's wrong out of pure habit? Do you discuss your problems with others in a constructive attempt to solve them? Or are you just venting and re-inforcing negativity in the process?

A number of years ago a friend introduced me to Deborah, a very pessimistic woman who, to her credit, was determined to change her negative ways. She told me the day we met that she had devised an experiment to get rid of her negativity. It was one of the simplest experiments I've ever heard of. She decided that she would write the words "Drop the negativity and focus on the blessings" on three-by-five index cards. She would carry one card in her purse, tape one to the visor in her car, and tape another to her refrigerator. Every time a negative thought crept into her mind, she would read the card.

Several months later she glowingly told me about the early results. When her old habit surfaced, she would look at the index card and repeat the words. After a while, she noticed that her negative attitude was beginning to change.

After six months Deborah and I bumped into each other again. The transformation was astonishing. She claimed to be one of the most genuinely positive people she knew. Speaking with her, I could sense she was right. She said that changing her habit of negativity was one of the easiest things she had ever done and doing so had changed her life forever.

We all have the power to reduce the percentage of time we spend focused on what's wrong and spend that time appreciating what's right instead. You will be amazed at how rewarding this shift in thinking can be. By focusing on the blessings, you will become more easily satisfied, loving, grateful, and appreciative.

As negative thoughts creep into your mind, learn to let them pass and replace them with thoughts about all that's right instead. The best part of this change is that all it takes is a little bit of intent, practice, and repetition.

15.

A GOLDEN PAUSE

My wife, Kris, and I attended a life-changing weekend meditation seminar a few years ago in Oakland, California. The highlight of the seminar was a series of short, unannounced breaks the organizers called "golden pauses."

These pauses took place approximately every hour and a half, lasted five to ten minutes, and were wonderfully received by everyone in the room. A pleasant little bell would ring and signal the beginning of the break. All at once, everyone in the room—hundreds of us—became calm. We stopped talking and dropped everything we were doing. We were instructed to sit in comfortable positions, to breathe and focus on the beauty of the breath, and to simply relax. It was a time to be still, quiet, and calm and appreciate the fact that we were alive.

Whenever Kris and I go to a workshop, we try to take something away that will stay with us for a long time. The idea of golden pauses has stuck like Velcro! We have found that golden pauses have the power to make the most impossible day manageable by giving us the perspective we need to get through it. Many times I have been angry or irritated at someone in my family on returning home from a long plane trip. Kris will smile at me and say that it's time for a golden pause. She takes out a little bell we got just for this purpose, she rings it, and we pause for just a few minutes. This little break invariably interrupts my negative thinking and readjusts my mental attitude. It's such an easy yet powerful way to change the course of a day.

A golden pause allows you to interrupt any moment —morning, noon, or night—when you feel tired, overwhelmed, or irritated and infuse it with positive energy. For me, it's a plane trip that can put me in a bad mood. For others, I know it's a long commute or a hard day at the office. A five-minute golden pause (or even a two-minute pause if that's all the time you have) usually reverses all of that negativity and then some.

But you don't have to be tired or irritated to benefit. A golden pause can make a day that's already wonderful even more glorious. Often Kris and I are having a completely peaceful day and one of us will suggest a golden pause just to focus on and appreciate the joy we are feeling. The pause reinforces and deepens feelings we are already having.

I once mentioned the concept of golden pauses during a lecture on the East Coast. Several months later I met a man at another lecture in Las Vegas who had been in the East Coast audience that day. Steve came up to say hello after my talk and shared with me the following story.

Steve referred to himself as having been an "overreactive hothead." During a particularly stressful time in his business, someone took advantage of the lack of business experience on the part of one of Steve's employees. He said that when this happened, he was about to lose it. I asked him what losing it meant for him. Steve explained that it might have meant a physical fight, a lawsuit, or, at the very least, a huge embarrassing scene in front of lots of people.

But in that moment of great stress, he said some part of him remembered the notion of the golden pause. Why he chose this instant to give it a try we'll never know, but he did. Instead of losing it that day, Steve imagined a tiny bell ringing, signaling the beginning of a golden pause.

He immediately began paying attention to all that he had to be grateful for. His mind became clear. His body relaxed, and he felt calmer. He started to breathe in and out several times and to appreciate the gift of breath. According to Steve, the golden pause went on for about five minutes, after which time he imagined a bell ringing again to signal the end of the break.

When it was over, he said, his body language was entirely different. He was relaxed and calm. Fighting or causing a scene was the furthest thing from his mind. He handled the situation calmly and professionally, and the problem never arose again.

I often practice a golden pause when the day seems to be speeding up too quickly or when life seems to be overwhelming. Golden pauses have a way of transforming my relationship to the world. Once the pause is over, I see the world and everyone in it quite differently.

A golden pause might take only a few minutes of your time, but the change in you will be substantial, quantifiable, and lasting.

So give the golden pause technique a try. It's easy and very relaxing, and it can be done virtually anywhere. Golden pauses alter your entire perspective on life, teaching you the value and wisdom of a calm, quiet mind. Golden pauses are one of the highlights of my day, and I hope they will become so for you as well. In fact, why not begin right now? *Ding!*

16.

PLANT A SEED OF DOUBT

A friend of mine enjoys listening to talk radio. He said that although he often finds the advice and commentary sound, what he finds distasteful is the certainty with which the hosts present their points of view. Whether they are on the left or right politically, whether they are social liberals or social conservatives, isn't the issue. The issue for him is that the hosts come across as arrogant, self-righteous, and rigid in their positions. They have zero doubt that their way is right and everyone else is wrong. There couldn't possibly be any other way.

As I look back on my life and think of all the people I've known, those who have been the least happy and the most hostile were those who couldn't see the two sides to an issue. Or they couldn't comprehend that someone else might see the world differently. Conversely, people who are able to see that the world is not always black and white and who understand that "our way" is not the "only way" are almost always the kindest, most tolerant, happiest, and easiest people to be around.

Please know that I'm not advocating becoming someone who can't take a stance, defend a position, or stand up for what's right or protest against what's wrong. There's a time and place for all of this. Instead, what I'm suggesting is that you plant a seed of doubt in your mind. Maybe, just maybe, there is another side to the argument.

One of my best friends, Jim, is a great supporter of the art of debate. Years ago he was the captain of his university's debate team and an outstanding debater. Each year Jim invites me to one of the nation's fiercest rivalries, the debates between the University of California at Berkeley and Stanford. I've been attending these debates for several years now, and I've been surprised at what I've learned in the process.

Perhaps the most eye-opening experience I have had as a result of witnessing these top-level debates is the realization that there really are two sides to an argument. What amazes me about good debaters is that they are capable of choosing which side of the argument to defend by the flip of a coin.

In other words, as often as not, good debaters would rather be arguing the other side. And they could do it just as articulately. Before you read on, think about that for a moment. The ramifications are important. The flexibility of debaters shows us that there is always a good argument to counter our position no matter how dearly we hold it.

When you listen to a debate, you often find yourself listening to an argument and then nodding in agreement. Just when you think you've made up your mind, suddenly the other side makes a point that is so clever and makes so much sense that you find yourself changing your position. I never knew I could be so wishy-washy and full of doubt until I went to a Cal-Stanford debate.

Make a habit of planting a seed of doubt in your own mind about how much you know something to be true. Planting a seed of doubt doesn't mean that you have to force yourself to believe something you don't—you're simply opening your mind to the possibility that there's be a different perspective to consider. Once you admit this to yourself, the enormous pressure you may have felt always to prove you are right is lifted. An open mind is essential for true happiness. So plant a seed of doubt and see what grows.

17.

BELIEVE IT OR NOT, THIS TOO SHALL PASS

I don't know how to describe this change other than to say that one day a few weeks ago I woke up on the wrong side of the bed. It was just one of those days. From the moment I woke up I was grumpy, frustrated, and angry. I snapped at my kids as they got ready for school. My fuse was short.

My daughter Jazzy, who has learned to not take bad moods (her own or others) as seriously or personally as she used to, offered some comfort and advice as I drove her to school. She said, "Dad, I think you're in a bad place today."

I immediately snapped back with my classic response when in a horrible mood: "No, I'm not."

"Okay, you're right, Dad," she said, "but can I give you some advice anyway?"

"I guess," I replied, trying to be respectful.

She said, "I'd try to take it easy today, and if at all possible, don't make any big decisions. Return as few calls as you can, and whatever you do, stay away from your e-mail. Trust me, Dad, things will look better tomorrow, maybe even in a few hours. Why don't you go take a walk or spend some time with Ty [our golden retriever]." And with that, she kissed me on the cheek, opened the door, and walked away toward school.

As I drove toward my office I reflected on what my daughter had said. My, how things had changed. I must have given her the same pep talk over a hundred times, and here she was giving it back to me. I couldn't help smiling, which immediately helped me recognize that she was right.

Nothing in my life had changed since the day before, and today my life had suddenly become unbearable. The simple and sole explanation? My mood had plummeted.

That was it. That was all I needed to know. No fancy psychobabble or sophisticated explanations needed. There was no need to visit a therapist, figure anything out, or change anything in my life.

What I had forgotten myself was something I had been telling others for years: be aware that your mood is the *starting place* of your experience, not the *end product*. In other words, a bad mood (or even a good one) colors the way you see things, so it is important to be aware that you might need to make adjustments. When you're in a bad mood, everything in your life— your family, your job, your home, your past, your friends, your physical fitness, your financial security— is going to seem inadequate. Any of these things will seem to present a legitimate reason to become upset—but none of them really do, because none of them have changed. Remember that yesterday, when you were in a better place emotionally, these very same aspects of life were cause for celebration. So it's your mood that determines your moment-to-moment state of mind.

Once you realize the unbelievable power that a bad mood has to convince you that your life is worse than it really is, you can make certain allowances until your mood improves—which it inevitably will. You can, as my daughter suggested to me, avoid making important decisions when you're low, angry, or stressed out. And even if you must make a decision during one of these times, at least you can be aware that your mood may be tainting your judgment.

You can postpone getting back to people, you can take a walk, or you can at least take some deep breaths. But most important, you can simply be aware that your mood is low and avoid trying to figure it out. In fact, in my opinion, that's the worst thing you can do. Why? When you're in a bad mood, you'll come up with dozens of reasons why you're feeling down. You'll blame everything and everyone from your parents, friends, and kids to your job, the government, society, and anything else you can think of.

Remember (and this is key): if you feel it's really critical to take care of a problem when you're in a bad place, that problem will surely still be there when your mood improves. And the same things that seemed so dreadful and urgent will once again seem just fine and more manageable.

EASIER THAN YOU THINK

This small adjustment in your awareness can and will make a world of difference in the quality of your life. Knowing a mood is just a mood will save you from making some horrible mistakes and maybe from embarrassing yourself and having to apologize later. I only wish they would teach this in school!

18.

SET YOUR EXPECTATIONS TO ZERO

Set your expectations to zero? "What," you might ask, "are you talking about?" I've made this suggestion to audiences before, and I've heard a number of gasps. People naturally wonder why, as a motivational speaker, I seem to be telling them to have no motivation. But once they hear my logic, they usually relax and fall in love with the idea.

Before I tell you what I mean by setting your expectations to zero, let me explain what I *don't* mean. I absolutely, positively am not talking about letting go of your dreams or goals, not working hard, not believing in yourself, or not having tremendous perseverance.

I believe in high standards, and I believe we all benefit from having high standards for ourselves and for others. I also think it's important to pick yourself up when you fall down and to try again even harder the second time. I also believe in competition and that without it our modern lives would be far less comfortable and enjoyable. Competition is one of the factors that motivates us to achieve and perform. And motivation *is* good.

Okay, so what do I mean when I say set your expectations to zero?

I first heard this idea from a dear friend of my dad's who died about a year ago. Wally was without a doubt one of the happiest and most satisfied people I ever met. In all the years I knew him, which was for most of my life, I never once heard him complain about anything. He never spoke ill of another human being and never wished his life were different than it was. And while he had a lot less than almost everyone I knew, he had a richer life on the *inside,* where it really matters.

I remember asking him about his grounded and optimistic approach to life in his later years, while he was fighting cancer (and still not complaining), and here is what he said: "Richard, when I look in the mirror, I set my expectation to zero. That way, everything I see is a miracle. I've lived my entire life that way, and it's always kept me happy and peaceful."

Indeed it did, right up until the day he died.

Do you see how you can both try hard and persevere and yet, at the same time, keep your expectation level in check? You can work out in the gym, for example, and still, when you look in the mirror, set your expectations to zero. That way, you appreciate the body you have been given, as opposed to resenting it and wishing it were different. It's an entirely new way of living and of looking at life. Even at the very end of Wally's life, he would say, "Life doesn't get any better than this. I have today. I have my friends. I can breathe. I'm alive. I'm very happy to be here." And the most beautiful part of Wally's attitude was that everyone who knew him knew that he meant every single word.

When you're disappointed in life, it's virtually always because what you're experiencing isn't matching up to what you were expecting the experience to be. When you think about it, what you are expecting is at least partially something you've made up as you move along through life. You imagine that life is going to be a certain way, and when it isn't, you feel disappointed. What Wally figured out was that it was better to set his expectations to zero than to make up a life that was bound to disappoint him. It sure worked for him, and I'm finding that it's working for me too.

Here are just a few examples of how expectations—either of some aspect of our own performance or that of someone else—can cause us pain or make us unhappy or depressed.

How about if you weigh 140 pounds and your goal is to weigh 132 pounds in one month's time? You psychologically invest in your success and tell yourself over and over, "I can do it." Well, you probably can. But suppose you step on the scale after thirty days and it says 139, or even 141? What now? Do you beat yourself up psychologically, say mean things to yourself, berate yourself, and so forth? If so, *what* caused the disappointment? Again, it was the expectation. There was absolutely nothing wrong with making the effort to lose weight—it may have been healthy and even fun—but the expectation that the result had to be a certain way was doomed to create disappointment unless, of course, the result exactly matched or exceeded your expectation.

Suppose you work hard for a reputable company. The company is under no legal obligation to reward its best employees with year-end bonuses, but it's understood that such bonuses are paid. You, believing that you're one of the best, spend November guessing how much your bonus is going to be. You aren't sure of the amount, but you have a pretty good idea. Then in December you go on a spending spree with your credit cards in anticipation of your bonus.

Unfortunately, this year the company didn't do as well and decides not to hand out bonus checks to anyone, even to its top people. Needless to say, you are crushed, hurt financially, and embarrassed, all because of one thing—expectation.

Setting your expectations for yourself and for others as close to zero as you possibly can is easier than you think, but it does take practice. If you can do this, however, you will eliminate a great deal of future disappointment that could result from things not turning out the way you wished they would.

Remember: lowering your expectations absolutely does not mean that you should stop working hard or encouraging your loved ones to slack off. It simply means that, once you've done all you can, you completely let go of your expectations of the outcome. If you can do this, you will have eliminated one of the single greatest sources of stress and disappointment known to mankind. And you will have found one of the keys to a lifetime of happiness.

19.

ARE YOU IN THERE?

Jessica was only eight years old, but certainly old enough to know that something was missing. I heard her say once in a group of other kids her age, "My parents are there, but sometimes it's like they aren't there."

For a moment think about what it's like when you're talking to someone and it's really obvious that he isn't paying attention to what you're saying. Instead, he's looking at his watch or glancing past your shoulder. You look in his eyes and they're absent. When this has happened to me, I've even found myself silently asking the question, "Are you in there?" You can tell there are many places this person would rather be. You feel no connection.

This lack of presence is annoying when you're an adult; it's painful when you're a child—especially when the person's eyes you're looking into are those of your own parent.

Now think for a moment what it's like to be with someone who *is* really there with you—who listens to you, fully present, engaged in the conversation, happy to be right where he or she is. When you talk to people like this, you can tell there is no place they would rather be. Being with someone like that is so refreshing, encouraging, and reassuring. It feels safe, even magical. Truly one of the highlights of being alive is sharing that kind of connection.

In addition to making those you're with feel slighted and unimportant, "not being present" takes its toll on you as well. It's exhausting and frustrating to have a busy mind that can't remain calm and present in one place. A mind that can't stay still is usually anxious and easily bothered.

On the other hand, someone who is able to stay centered and present feels the benefits that come along with that state of mind. He or she is able to be calm and focused most of the time. A person with a mind that doesn't randomly run wild is less inclined to create internal drama and doesn't tend to blow things out of proportion. These are two very important ingredients of inner peace.

The most surprising thing of all is that the difference between someone who is present and someone who is not isn't as significant as you might think. In fact, all it takes to make the shift from one state of mind to the other is—you guessed it—a small change in your intent and some follow-up practice to reinforce that change.

The small change you're looking for is learning how to consciously choose to keep your mind and your focus on the one conversation or activity you are engaged in at the moment. Step forward and offer your full and absolute concentration. If you are talking to your child, for example, try to think of nothing else, no matter what it is, even for just five or ten minutes. Similarly, when you're with anyone else, make that person feel as though he or she is the most important person in the world to you at that moment.

In a nutshell, that is essentially all there is to it. This is the art of being present. If your mind wanders (which it will do, especially at first), quietly remind yourself to come back to the conversation or the activity. Drop the rest of your thinking, or any other business, knowing that you can come back to it later. Nothing is more important than what you are doing right now.

If you are engaged in a project at work or at home, do your best to focus on nothing else. Get in the habit of doing one thing at a time and, more important, not allowing your mind to wander. This is tough to do in today's world, and staying focused is certainly the exception, not the norm. However, you'll be amazed at how efficient you'll become and how joyful each activity and conversation will be.

The easiest part about becoming more present is that each day will present you with an unlimited number of opportunities to practice. You can take the most mundane activity and turn it into an opportunity to practice being more present. Two things I love to do, for example, are watering the plants in the summer and sweeping the yard. Both activities are like meditations for me. While I do them, I keep my mind as clear as possible and simply sweep or water—nothing else. When a thought enters my mind, I allow it to drift away.

I think of both activities as relaxation and practice times, so that the next time I'm with Kris, or one of my daughters, or a friend, or someone I work with, or even a stranger, I might be just a little bit more present. The first time someone says to you, "Thank you for just being there for me, for just listening," you'll feel on top of the world. The most amazing part of all is that you didn't have to "do" anything to get there. Instead, you were able to be present to this person by *not* doing certain things—like filling your mind with other stuff that was unrelated to what was going on in the moment.

Without question, this is an example of a small change paying huge dividends for yourself and for everyone you come into contact with. By becoming more present, you'll experience better communication, increased productivity, better relationships, and greater peace of mind. With a little bit of practice, no one will be asking, "Are you in there?" It will be obvious that you are!

20.

FIND A WAY TO LAUGH
EVERY DAY

One day not too long ago, I was taking everything really seriously. It was one of those days when it was me against the world. I was overwhelmed, tired, and grumpy. Although it seemed like dozens of people were furious at me for a variety of reasons, the truth was that there were only a few people who were moderately irritated at me. It was my state of mind that was exaggerating everything, blowing it out of proportion.

As usual, my wife, Kris, had the perfect solution. We were sitting in the car together in a parking lot, and I was feeling sorry for myself. She said in a loving voice, "Richard, I'll give you five dollars if you can look at yourself in the mirror for an entire minute and not break into a laugh."

My initial instinct was that it would be the easiest five dollars I ever earned. But boy was I wrong. Peering into the rearview mirror, I lasted about five seconds before I saw how ridiculous I looked with a big frown on my face. Within a few seconds I was smiling, and soon after I started to laugh so hard that tears were streaming down my face. When Kris actually asked for the money, I couldn't stop laughing and my stomach started to hurt.

I heard once that it takes far more muscles to frown than it does to smile. I also know that when you smile, it's far more difficult to be depressed or even upset. Smiling and laughter are good medicine, no matter how you look at it.

We need to see the value in laughter instead of dismissing it as something frivolous or reserving it for good times. Once we see it in this light, we'll recognize that there are many ways to get there. If I can simply look at my own frown in the mirror and start laughing within a matter of seconds, imagine how easy it will be for you to come up with creative ways to make yourself laugh.

Friends of mine who need to laugh spend time with little kids—that usually works, since kids almost always bring a smile to your face. Or you can read a funny book, or watch your favorite comedy. I can turn on a rerun of any number of funny shows and usually be laughing within minutes. Laughing gets my mind off whatever it is that I'm taking too seriously.

Certainly, there are times when it's appropriate and imperative to deal with important issues in a serious way. However, when being serious brings you to the point of being overwhelmed, anxious, depressed, and despondent, any decisions you make are most likely not going to be good. Laughter is one of the best remedies when we have started taking things too seriously.

Whether at work or at home, when you've lost your sense of humor, you have lost your perspective as well. The act of laughing serves as a powerful reset button and restores the big-picture outlook. Laughing is our mind's way of telling us that everything can and will be okay. When we laugh, our bodies release molecules called endorphins that immediately make us start feeling better. Simply put, laughing is the easiest and most natural way we have of feeling better immediately.

It's certainly true that much of life needs to be taken very seriously. However, that doesn't mean we need to lose our sense of humor. On the contrary, the healing power of laughter is all the more reason to maintain and foster laughter in our lives. So find at least one reason to laugh today, tomorrow, and every day. You'll be glad you did, now and forever.

TURNING

on a

DIME

————————

21.

TURNING ON A DIME

One of the greatest signs of maturity—and incidentally, one of the secrets of happiness—is to know that the world and the vast majority of the people in it are not going to change. Simply put, we cannot expect the world to become more accommodating, nor can we assume that other people will eventually come around to our way of thinking. If anyone is going to change, it's going to have to be us. On the surface changing ourselves might seem like a tall order, but in reality all it takes is a small shift in the way we approach our relationships with others and with the world at large. All we need is a little insight and the willingness to be honest about our own habits.

One of the most exciting aspects of being human is that we have the inner resilience to change our habits at a moment's notice—we have the capacity to "turn on a dime." None of us is right all of the time. All of us make mistakes, use poor judgment, or get caught in ruts. The good news is that these patterns and decisions are not permanent. We are flexible.

Take the case of Evan, who had been married to his wife, Paula, for more than a decade. Their marriage was not in good shape. Evan had a horrible habit of interrupting virtually everyone, especially Paula. As a result, Paula had been resenting him for years. After losing two jobs (for not paying attention to his bosses or the directives being given to him), Evan sought help for both his job situation and his marriage.

After just a few sessions the therapist was able to help Evan recognize his pattern of incessant interruption. To his credit, Evan realized that he needed to alter his behavior. With this change of heart, he was able to turn on a dime and break free of a lifelong tendency that had been holding him back in all areas of life. By identifying his own habit, he was able immediately to become a better listener, and he began to interrupt others far less frequently. He fell into his old pattern from time to time but caught himself earlier and earlier in the process.

Paula appreciated the effort Evan put into this change in his behavior. As their communication improved, their marriage started showing signs of life. The negative cycle had been broken. Evan's change didn't take a magic wand or years of expensive therapy—in fact, it took only three sessions. But more important, what it took was an open mind and a willingness to make the change. In a matter of months Evan had saved his marriage and was well on his way to getting a new job.

If you've ever had the experience of saying to yourself, "I'm just not going to do that anymore," and you followed through with your internal commitment, then you've had the experience of turning on a dime.

We all have this capacity to turn on a dime and to change our lives for the better. We can change our relationship to individuals, as Evan did with his wife and his bosses, or to groups, such as our coworkers, friends, or customers. This change can take a variety of forms, such as communicating better, becoming more willing to compromise, reaching out, or becoming more humble.

Turning on a dime can also happen on a more global scale as we develop a better relationship with ourselves and with the world in general. We can become more tolerant and respectful of the ways in which others approach life. We can attempt to build rather than burn bridges.

Our capacity to turn on a dime is unlimited, and the best part is that we hold all the cards. It's empowering to know that by stepping forward with confidence you have the inner resources you need to make this happen. Knowing you have this capacity makes it all the more likely that it's going to happen to you— and soon.

22.

LAY OUT THE WELCOME MAT

My friend Marvin is a successful real estate developer. Marvin came up with a compassionate and creative idea for one of his new apartment projects. He felt that many competing developments were kid-unfriendly in very unnecessary ways. For example, communal areas were off limits to children for noise reasons during standard playtimes before and after school. Another policy that irked him was the one requiring that parents buy and replace any communal toys their child may have broken. To Marvin, this policy was not only too harsh but bad for business. Toys most often get broken over time, and the expense to the apartment owner is so minimal that this policy comes across as cheap and mean-spirited.

Marvin had the manager of one of his apartment buildings post the following sign in the children's recreation area. It read, "Kids, please be careful with the toys. But if you break something, don't worry—we were kids once ourselves."

The manager told my friend that the very first person to take a tour of the development after that sign was posted was a single mom with a five-year-old child. When the woman read the sign, a tear came to her eye and she said: "I don't even need to see any more of this place. I want to live here." Having one less vacancy at the apartment complex saved the owner about $10,000 a year. Needless to say, that was enough to replace the broken toys many times over. And all it took was a simple welcome.

When I heard Marvin's story, I immediately thought of many other possible benefits of being welcoming in everything from making business decisions to dealing with neighbors or people who are looking for help. When you are welcoming, you build up instant goodwill and rapport with people. It is a win-win situation for everyone involved.

To call laying out the welcome mat a small change is probably an overstatement. In fact, it's merely a tiny change in behavior. But the tiny change of becoming more welcoming can mean the difference between experiencing success or failure, making friends or foes, being seen as generous or cheap, or creating goodwill versus bad feelings. And last but certainly not least, being welcoming to others can mean the difference between feeling good about yourself or not.

The best news of all is that the change is well within your own power. So reach out to others and become more welcoming in whatever small way you can, whether it's by taking the NO TRESPASSING sign off your gate or bringing a casserole to a new neighbor. You and everyone around you will reap the rewards.

23.

A SMALL SECRET

Years ago my friend Roger's thirteen-year-old nephew was not performing well at school even though his standardized test scores were high and everyone knew he was an extremely bright kid. Roger met with Ben one Sunday morning and brought a one-page current events essay from a popular news magazine. Roger asked the boy to take a few minutes to read it and then asked him ten rather technical, factual questions that could be answered from the essay. His nephew got two correct and missed eight.

Roger then handed Ben ten flashcards with highlighted points from the article that he had prepared ahead of time and asked him to review the cards for a few minutes. When Roger asked Ben ten different questions about the same article, Ben got all of them correct.

It was a rather simple discovery for Ben, and one that I myself learned many years ago in college. Ben continued to use flashcards throughout his education and still uses them to this day. We can read and reread the same material without retaining the essential information. The flashcard is a simple and effective learning tool that enables us to grasp and retain information. Whether we are at school or at work, or maybe learning a language just for fun, using flashcards is an easy change that makes a big difference.

If you ever have to give a talk, whether at work or perhaps at an event such as a wedding, flashcards are an amazingly efficient way to keep calm and poised. By putting all the big ideas down on an index card, you can avoid the embarrassing possibility of forgetting your lines and you won't be criticized for reading.

By the way, Ben grew up to be a successful and happy businessman. In fact, the last I heard was that the C student was successfully practicing law in California and had received his graduate degree from the University of California at Berkeley, one of the top schools in the nation! One small change certainly made a world of difference in Ben's life.

24.

LEARN TO SAY NO

Over the last decade or so, I have been giving talks around the country to a lot of people from various walks of life. During this time I've taken dozens of informal surveys to discover what is the most frustrating aspect of our day-to-day lives. After talking with thousands of ordinary people, I'm now pretty sure I know the answer. The good news is that with a very small change, most of that frustration would disappear overnight.

When I ask people what frustrates them more than anything else, the most common answer is that there is just not enough time. From having too much to do to feeling burdened with commitments to experiencing constant daily stress, the number-one complaint boiled down to simply not having enough time in the day. This begs the question: why don't we have enough time?

Part of the answer is that humans are naturally inclined to want to help each other. Think about it. None of us would be here today if we had not received a great deal of assistance from those around us. We help others because it is part of our makeup and because helping others feels good. So what's the problem? Well, this instinct for offering a hand, time, and assistance can lead to our lives being overwhelmed. Here's how.

We live in a culture filled with addictions. We're addicted to all sorts of things, including alcohol, drugs, money, great bodies, youth, sex, perfect abs, gambling, television, movies, shopping, spending, work, sugar, upward mobility, achievement, and faster service. We're even addicted to being right, improving ourselves, and being famous or recognized. Often the underlying problem is our culture's assumption that more is better. Indeed, most of us cross the line to the point of excess in some part of our lives. For example, if your goal is to be a good person, you might believe that volunteering is a good idea. And it may well be. But how much volunteering should you do? Five hours a week? Ten? Twenty? Thirty?

If your goal is to be in great physical shape, you may join the gym. This is a great idea. But should you work out thirty minutes a day? How about an hour? What about two? Why not three? You can see that given our cultural adherence to the "more is better" philosophy, many of us soon develop huge problems.

So how does our natural inclination to help, which is a positive trait, become negatively affected by this cultural addiction? Combining the "more is better" attitude with our innate human desire to be helpful leads us directly to the number-one frustration we have about daily life—not enough time. We say yes to things when we are already overwhelmed and would rather say no. We are in the habit of believing that more is better, and so instead of saying no, we agree and take on additional responsibilities we have no time for.

If we continue to follow this pattern, how are we ever going to downsize our schedules? Our entire lives are affected by this addiction to continually doing more. We're so busy running from one activity to the next, just to cross things off the list, that the quality of what we do is often compromised. Being in this state can easily make us feel like victims, even though we are the ones who have robbed ourselves of free time.

The only way out of this mess is to admit that we played a part in its creation. But we shouldn't be too hard on ourselves. We *can* clean up the mess.

It's funny that a word as small as "no"—just two letters—can be so powerful. But it is. And to get out of your mess, you're going to have to start using it much more often.

To begin with, take an honest look at your schedule. Look carefully at all of your so-called obligations. Why are you on this committee or on that board? Do you *have* to be? Do you *want* to be? What about all those weekly meetings? Are they necessary? Be honest. You may love some of your commitments, or all of them. Or you might be attending at least some meetings or groups out of a commitment you made years ago that no longer fits your interests or needs. What about the volunteer positions? Maybe one or even two nourish your soul—but three? You can't truly make a difference if you are constantly overwhelmed and exhausted. You need to be honest with yourself. Do you have time for all these commitments, and are they necessary given your current life circumstances?

It doesn't take much of a change to start feeling less overwhelmed. The usual objection is that getting out of a commitment is going to hurt someone's feelings. Well, that's just something we're going to have to get over.

Kris walked into a nonprofit company board meeting recently having decided to resign. Her biggest concern was that her decision would be taken the wrong way. The truth was that her commitment was overwhelming her. She loved the company, and she shared those sentiments when she told the members of the board that she needed to quit. She explained that she fully intended to stay involved in less labor-intensive ways. In a one-hour meeting Kris was able to get herself out of a huge time commitment that had been hanging over her head. She was honest about her feelings and felt good about her decision. You'll find that when you back away from things for the right reasons, most people will respect you for it. In fact, they may wish they had the courage to do the very same thing.

The way to eliminate the problem of having limited time is to learn to say no to new requests. I'm not suggesting that you never say yes, only that you look after your time very carefully. Remember that you have the ability to fix what is for most of us our number-one frustration. Get in the habit of saying no. It may be difficult at first, but it gets easier with practice.

There is nothing wrong in making sure that you have time to live your life without feeling overwhelmed. It is your right. So start enjoying more time in your day-to-day life. Experience some true peace of mind and perhaps some free time. It is all possible with that little two-letter word—no.

25.

STOP THE BLAME GAME

Over the years I've tried to figure out the difference between happy people and miserable people, between optimists and pessimists, between those who are generally relaxed and accepting about life versus those who are stressed and resentful. Though I believe there are a number of determining factors, one that can't be emphasized enough is the tendency of those who are happy not to blame others for their unhappiness or misfortune. In other words, happy people take responsibility for what happens in their lives—the good *and* the bad.

Here's an example of how that slight shift in perspective can make a world of difference. David was an unhappy guy who was always blaming someone else for his problems. At work he was quick to point the finger at colleagues when his projects did not meet expectations. When David had issues with his neighbors, it was always their fault. And when he and his wife were bickering, she was always misguided. He even blamed the painter when he didn't like the way the color turned out on his house—despite the fact that he was the one who had chosen and provided the paint!

Nothing was ever his fault.

After David's marriage failed—which of course wasn't his fault either—his life began to fall apart. Eventually he hit bottom and began to search for answers. After listening to the advice of one of his childhood friends, David started to look inward.

For the first time in his life David was taking a step forward and examining his own contribution to the problems in his life. This was in sharp contrast to his pattern of placing the blame on anyone and everyone but himself.

David said that making this shift was "like taking a two-hundred-pound weight off my shoulders." Instead of insisting that the world behave according to his every wish (which it had never done) and being resentful that the world wouldn't give him exactly what he wanted, he started instead to take a look at what *he* was doing and what he might be able to do differently. Instead of blaming everyone around him—his neighbors, his kids, his ex-wife, his friends, his colleagues— he tried to put himself in their shoes. All of a sudden, he could see things from an entirely new perspective.

Here's an example of this significant change. David's neighbor Jeff had been complaining for years about two old trucks sitting in David's yard. David resented Jeff for complaining and had been bad-mouthing him behind his back to anyone who would listen.

But after he had his insight about not blaming others, David decided to take control of this ongoing feud. He walked up to Jeff's house, something that had never occurred to him to do before. And even before he knocked on the door, when he looked at his trucks from his neighbor's perspective, he could immediately see why Jeff had been upset for so long. The truth of the matter was that from his neighbor's perspective, the trucks were a legitimate eyesore.

The walk over to his neighbor's house had taken about sixty seconds. Yet David's stubbornness had prevented him from taking that sixty-second walk for more than ten years. Slightly embarrassed, David walked back home. He wrote an apology to his neighbor and promptly moved the trucks.

The small change of learning not to blame others will make an enormous difference in your life. When you blame others, you blind yourself to your own responsibility and also give up ownership of the effects of your decisions. When you consciously stop blaming others, you can take full control of your life, put old hurts behind you, and move forward with confidence and grace.

26.

BE CAREFUL WHAT
YOU DO AND SAY

How do our choices affect the people around us, and what do they teach us about ourselves? Especially for parents, bosses, or anyone in the position of being a role model, it is critical to pay close attention to these choices, which have a direct effect on others.

Think about it. Everything we do has the potential to influence another human being. This potential increases when we are in a position of authority. Parents who refuse to eat healthy food at the dinner table directly affect their child's relationship to food. A boss who decides that making money is more important than being ethical directly affects every single employee in the company. From big decisions like these to smaller everyday decisions, such as walking away from a family member during an argument, our choices have consequences.

The key element here is not to second-guess yourself but rather to become conscious of how your life choices influence those around you. This small change in awareness will have a potent impact on your life.

Here are a few specific questions for parents that illustrate the ways in which both conscious and unconscious choices influence their children. Remember that there are no right or wrong answers to these questions—they are simply food for thought.

1. In your home, do you emphasize reading or television?
2. Do you spend money wisely? Do you discuss the value of a dollar?
3. Do you idolize and talk about great scholars or about great athletes?
4. Does your family engage in frequent arguments or do you practice compromise?

5. Do you talk about the way things look and place value on external appearances?

It should be clear from these questions that the daily choices we make can become a significant influence. This influence can be positive, and that is why it is so vital to be conscious of our actions.

Parents and family members certainly aren't the only influences in young people's lives. For example, you may emphasize the importance of saving a dollar at home, but your child may well be shaped by the runaway consumerism in our culture, which is outside your influence.

Even if you can't control all the influences on your children, however, you can help matters significantly by becoming aware of your own choices. But before you can modify or even eliminate some of these behaviors and choices, you must become aware of them.

My friend Sam used to brag to his teenage daughter Jessica that when he was in school he would wait until the night before an important exam to study. Despite this risky study habit, Sam had been able to pull off straight As. There was one small problem, however, with sharing this history with his daughter: while Jessica was extremely bright and capable of great grades, she couldn't do it by cramming. Jessica, like most kids, wanted to be just like her dad, but she needed to study the old-fashioned way—every night.

When a friend of Sam's pointed out the way in which he was negatively influencing his daughter, a lightbulb went off. He stopped offering positive reinforcement for her last-minute studying, and he learned not to repeat the problem with his son, who was only in the fifth grade. I thought this was an incredible example of the power of small changes.

Being aware of our own choices gives us the ability to have a positive influence on the people around us. But more than that, we also discover how others influence us in ways we hadn't realized.

27.

FIRST THINGS FIRST

When it comes to business, this is one of the simplest changes you can make. It takes very little effort. If you do make this change, it can make you more effective and productive, and as a direct result your life will become much easier.

Marsha is a successful businesswoman in the financial services industry. Like many successful people, she told me that she has been asked hundreds of times for the secret of her success.

Marsha said that her answer has always been the same. When I heard what it was, it didn't surprise me that her answer was not the obvious and pat one we usually hear: work hard. Instead, her answer is the same one offered by almost everyone I know who is successful.

What Marsha does is to focus her energy and time on what is most productive and potentially profitable. Marsha understands that her time is her most valuable resource. So before she spends it, she thinks about whether what she's about to spend time on is contributing to her goals—or not. In other words, she knows her priorities, and so her decisions are purpose-driven.

That's all there is to it. Before you brush this off as overly simplistic advice, consider what most of us do instead. We can be divided up into several categories.

First, there are those of us who tackle things as they come in, regardless of time-sensitivity or importance. The task might be potentially significant, such as making a call to a customer, or it might be mundane, such as filling out a report or answering a phone call. Those of us in this category don't discriminate at all. We approach demands on our time like the famous voice-mail recording, which always reminds us that we've been put on hold "in the order received."

Obviously those of us who handle work in this way

are just trying to stay on top of things. Yet, if you think about, demands come at us during any given day or week in a somewhat random way. When we handle work in this fashion, we spend our time on tasks that are most likely not priorities. Instead of consciously making choices and prioritizing, we let the outside world randomly dictate what we do in our day-to-day work.

In the second category are those of us who respond mostly to so-called emergencies. We have such a huge to-do list that when we look at it we decide to tackle only those tasks that seem most urgent. Again, we run into a similar problem. Something may seem urgent, but it may or may not have much to do with what's truly important. For example, in my business I could spend lots of time answering calls, mail, and e-mails, but if I never got around to writing, my books would never get done and there wouldn't be any phone calls or mail or e-mails to respond to. Like almost everyone I know, I could be busy up to twelve hours a day and never actually get to the most important tasks.

It is easy to rationalize putting out the fires at work, but it is absolutely critical to be aware of the bigger picture. The urgent stuff might keep us busy for months, and it is far too easy to lose sight of our larger professional goals.

There are of course other ways in which people prioritize their workloads. Some people choose to do what appears to be the easiest or least stressful. For example, if you're this kind of person, you may have an uncomfortable phone call to make that could secure a sale, as well as a couple of flyers or direct-mail pieces to send out. One task is simple and mindless, whereas the other is difficult and uncomfortable. Guess which you do first?

Finally, there are people who waste time with simple distractions. They spend a lot of time straightening their desks, making lists, returning less than productive phone calls, or sharpening pencils.

The small change is to alter your mind-set when it comes to your work life and put first things first. To do this, you have to know your goals and be really honest with yourself about your habits. Then you have to work to change the habits that are not serving your goals.

Before I reflected about this issue, I was someone who responded to things as they came in. It seemed extremely difficult to get work done, especially the work that was most important to me, like writing books. In 1996, with the help of a good friend, I saw my own habit. Everything changed. I started to get up early in the morning and start my day by focusing on writing. As old temptations arose, such as the desire to check my answering machine, go through my briefcase, or look at my calendar, I'd catch myself and bring my attention back to my first priority. After a while it became second nature to focus only on what was most relevant—what came first before everything else.

Since that time I've met hundreds of successful people who do essentially the same thing in their own fields. They do what they need to do in order to focus on what's most important and put first things first.

Again, this is a small shift in behavior that is worth its weight in gold. Try it today, and you'll see what I mean. This is a small change that could earn you a fortune, and I know it's one that can bring you more joy and satisfaction, because you'll spend more time on those things that really matter.

28.

INNOCENT UNTIL PROVEN GUILTY

The other day, while I was sitting on a bench waiting for BART (San Francisco's Bay Area Rapid Transit system), I overheard the following conversation between two women.

The first woman—let's call her Claire—was commiserating with another woman whom we'll call Ellen.

"Jane has gone too far," Claire said. "She's always stealing my ideas at work, but now she's even stealing my brilliant plan for John's birthday party."

Apparently Claire felt that Jane was going to use her idea and create essentially an identical birthday celebration for her own young son.

Claire went on. "Jane's driving me crazy. Can't she ever come up with anything on her own?"

Ellen chimed in. "If I were you, I'd give her a piece of my mind. Think of all the times she's stolen your ideas. It's time to confront her."

Sitting there listening, I couldn't help but feel a little saddened. These grown women sounded like angry teenagers. One of the mistakes both Claire and Ellen were making was assuming that if they could somehow prove Jane wrong, they would magically feel better. That's just not true. Think about the times you've put someone in their place or proven them wrong. You may have fantasized for weeks or months about how great it was going to be. But after the fact you were the one who felt terrible.

It's not always easy to take the high road when you feel you're being wronged. But remember, in the end you're the one who will reap the greatest reward. You'll end up happy. There are obvious things Claire could do in the future, such as not telling Jane her plans, but there was absolutely no need for her to spend even one moment being upset about what had taken place. Confronting Jane would not have solved the problem. You can imagine the scenario: after such a confrontation, every day at work would be more unpleasant than the one before.

The small shift is to change our intention. Instead of assuming that someone else is guilty of bad intentions, we need to assume their innocence. We can repeat the following words to ourselves: "My intention is to assume innocence and to trust in the goodwill of others. If, on occasion, others break this trust, it will not adversely affect my sense of well-being. If need be, I'll make adjustments, but I won't allow others to interfere with my personal happiness."

Suppose, like Claire, you have a great idea at work. But the next day when you show up, someone else has already shared the same idea. It's easy to assume that person stole your idea, but you have no proof. What you do have is two choices. You can assume the other party's guilt and expend endless energy feeling resentful and bitter, or you can assume it was a coincidence that someone else had your idea and let it go. This is a simple example of how assuming innocence can release negative feelings.

Many in our culture gossip as sport. For example,

we hear people regularly saying such things as, "He's missing so much work—I bet he's probably having an affair." We assume guilt when in reality this poor man's mother has been ill and he is spending less time at work to take care of her.

What is important to remember is that we are not giving up control or power by assuming the good nature of our fellow humans. Instead, we are taking control by not letting our assumptions run our lives.

Obviously if someone is acting in a way that has a negative effect on you directly, such as taking credit for your work, you have to take action. What this change addresses is the more frequent case of letting our imaginations and assumptions take over. The small change is a simple shift in intention. Assuming the best, not the worst, will result in an immediate improvement in your day-to-day life. Just think of all those negative thoughts you can start letting go of. It's hard to believe that a shift this small can be so powerful.

29.

NO MORE REGRETS

As I travel the country, I am always surprised by the number of people I meet who seem to be living with the constant burden of regret. I'm not talking about regrets about awful deeds such as murder or other crimes, but rather regrets over things that happen in the natural course of life that are over and done with. We waste so much energy and time feeling guilt or remorse about the past.

Some of what we regret can be changed, and some cannot. For example, there are people who regret the career choices they made years ago. Others regret that they didn't have children, or didn't have more children, and some even regret that they had children at all. Some regret that they haven't experienced more adventure in their lives, done more traveling, made more friends, changed jobs, taken more risks, been more charitable, and on and on it goes.

Every time we think and rethink and rethink again about something we regret, the emotional impact of our thoughts continues to grow. The more attention we pay to something, the harder it is to stop thinking about it. And this is why so many of us struggle with regrets. We get stuck in a cycle, and the regrets become increasingly difficult to dispose of.

It is in our best interest, however, to take a step forward and eliminate all the outstanding regret in our lives. Here's how you can do it.

Regret always has its orientation in the past. It's something you wish were different or something you wish you had handled differently. You may well want to make decisions in your life to remedy past mistakes if you can, but "crying over spilled milk" does not help.

Therefore, the way to eliminate regret is to commit to a new mind-set, one of forward motion. As thoughts that contain regret come up, the trick is to be aware of them and then let these thoughts go. Here's an example.

Suppose you're driving home, and a neighbor drives by with a nicer, more expensive car. A regretful thought enters your mind, such as, "I wish I had gone back to school and earned a degree so that I would have a better-paying job today." Instead of allowing that thought to percolate any further, say to yourself something like, "Ah-ha, no more regrets." It's okay to make light of it. After all, it was only a thought.

But here's where you reinforce the change you've just made. Follow up with a positive, life-affirming thought such as this: "I choose to believe that everything that has happened in my life happened for a reason. I have made good decisions that support a positive, wonderful life. I will not look back, unless it is to learn or appreciate something or to teach someone else a valuable life lesson."

To reiterate, the change to make regarding regrets is to first understand that regrets come from the past and that you can't go back in time. Second, you must realize that only you have the power to rid yourself of regret. You created it and now you must get rid of it.

All you need to do is to notice your thoughts of regret and catch them if you can. Drop these thoughts, knowing they are self-destructive and useless. And finally, give yourself a pep talk to reinforce your change, emphasizing that from this point forth, you will live in the present and look forward toward the future.

I promise you won't regret making this small change.

30.

LISTEN WITHOUT INTERRUPTING

A number of years ago I needed to solve a business problem I was experiencing. The issue was complex, and I was at the end of my rope trying to figure it out on my own. Luckily, friends of mine were kind enough to gather in my home to help me brainstorm some possible solutions. We sat around a large round table, and one by one my friends began dishing out their wisdom. Unfortunately, none of it was sinking in. For every piece of advice offered, I had an equally well thought out reason why that particular solution would not help me.

About an hour into our meeting, my dear friend

Michael suggested that we take a five-minute break. During the break he asked if he could speak to me privately. "So how do you think things are going so far?" he asked.

"Pretty good," I answered without much enthusiasm. Reflecting on how clever I was to be able to pick apart the ideas of such smart people, I added, "But I don't think we will be able to solve anything today."

"Why is that?" Michael asked.

"The issues are far too complicated to tackle at once," I responded. I suppose what I really thought was that there was no way anyone was clever enough to help solve these problems. I was, without knowing it, being a poor listener, not to mention arrogant and stubborn.

"Richard," Michael said in response, "I'd like to make a small suggestion that just might change your life. It's a tiny shift really, but I'll make the suggestion only with your permission and only if you're really interested in hearing what it is."

"Now you really have me curious," I told him. "Of course I want to hear what it is."

"All right, Richard. From now on, when anyone here is offering a suggestion, I want you to listen to

147

that person as if you were listening to music. Just let it in all the way. Don't offer any commentary on the suggestion, and no matter what you do, don't tell the person why the idea won't work. No interruptions whatsoever. The same holds true in your own mind, within your own thinking. Just listen quietly and allow the suggestions to sink in. Don't do anything with the suggestions just yet. Allow them to percolate for a while. If a disagreeable thought enters your mind, just let it go. Agreed?"

"Agreed," I said, feeling a little foolish as I realized that I hadn't really been listening to any of my friends for the previous hour.

Michael went on to explain that, "when you start to critique what is being said *while* it's being said, instead of just listening, your own biases, judgments, and ideas get in the way. They prevent you from learning anything new."

This was an eye-opening experience for me. I had always thought I was an above-average listener, but that day I learned to truly listen, and it was the beginning of a whole new life for me. What made me listen to Michael's suggestion that day instead of dismissing it or becoming defensive was that I could tell by the tone of his voice that he had my best interests at heart. After all, he was there on his own time to help me. He and my other friends had been through similar business situations dozens of times and knew so much more than I did on the subject. It was I who needed them, not the other way around.

It wasn't just the importance of listening that "clicked" for me that day. I also realized that at the same time I needed to be willing to consider the advice without dismissing it or interrupting the advice-giver. I understood that day that there is no advantage to interrupting or mentally critiquing someone who is giving you advice. After all, you can always consider the advice and decide later to not accept it.

I took Michael's advice, and within a few weeks the complex business problem was solved. More important, I had learned to start listening to people on a deeper level. My learning curve has skyrocketed since that time.

When you listen with a quieter mind to your loved ones, coworkers, educators, or anyone else with whom it's crucial that you really hear what's being said, both you and the person you're listening to will sense a world of difference. It feels good to listen, and it feels good to be listened to. Can you imagine how different the world might be if friends, husbands and wives, and even political leaders could listen to each other in this way?

One of the most beautiful aspects of this type of listening is its simplicity. It's more about what you *don't* do than about what you have to do. That's why I categorize it as a small change. All you have to do is ignore the noise in your mind while others are speaking to you and bite your tongue when you're tempted to jump in. You won't believe how much you will learn by just being quiet and listening.

31.

SAVE FOR A RAINY DAY!

I was standing behind a man in line at a coffee shop early one morning when he ordered his favorite drink, a large double mocha with whipped cream.

Waiting for our orders, we chatted for a while. I found out a few interesting things about this man, as he was quite talkative. First of all, his name was Tom, and he lived down the street. He told me that he had not one but two of these delicious coffee drinks five days a week—one before work and one on his way home. He considered the coffees his treat to himself. The cost each time was a whopping four dollars.

I also found out that although he was thirty-five years old, he had virtually no savings to his name.

(Don't ask how the subject came up—as I said, he was talkative.) He said the reason for his lack of savings was that at the end of each month he simply had no money left over. "I live paycheck to paycheck," he lamented.

This man was a perfect candidate for what I call the rainy day fund mentality, a technique of looking for small ways you can easily cut everyday expenses and invest them toward your future. All that's required is a small adjustment in mind-set, along with a little discipline to implement the idea.

Consider the double mocha this man was about to purchase. If he were simply to substitute a plain one-dollar coffee for one of his four-dollar mochas each day, he could still enjoy the one mocha *and* have three dollars per day to invest in savings. I'm no math wiz, but I believe the annual savings on that change alone, assuming a 240-workday year, would be $720, and if invested over twenty years at 8 percent, the value of that money would be $32,949. You have to admit, that's no small change! And if he could stand to switch to plain coffee altogether, his savings over time would be far more substantial.

Sometimes people decide to do the very same thing with their lunch savings. It's easy to get into the habit of going out to lunch at work and spending eight dollars a day, maybe even more, at a local restaurant. So if you're one of those people who usually spend forty dollars a week for lunch (and if you go out often, you know I'm being conservative in these estimates), what could happen if you started bringing your lunch to work instead? Suppose it cost you only three dollars to make your lunch instead of eight dollars to go out. This means you'd save five dollars a day to put into your rainy day fund. Here's the math. Five dollars each day for 240 workdays is $1,200. If you were to invest this money and could again earn 8 percent for twenty years, it would be worth $54,914!

Of course there are many other clever ways to save. If you can pay just one additional payment on your mortgage each year, you can save thousands of dollars (maybe even a lot more than that, depending on the size of your mortgage) and pay off your mortgage years sooner. I know a woman who figured her car payment for a new car would be around five hundred dollars per month if she financed the purchase through traditional means. She decided instead to postpone buying the new car for a few years and set up her own car fund. She opted to drive her old car until she had saved the money for a new one. She started putting exactly five hundred dollars a month into an investment account until she had saved the amount she needed to pay for the car in cash.

She figured that she saved tons of interest and didn't have any financial pressure to make payments. As soon as she bought the car, she simply started making additional payments into her car fund for any maintenance down the road and for her next car.

You might call any one of these ideas a small change, but you can see that in reality they add up to some really big money. And again, these are just a few ideas. Imagine all the ways you could save and invest if you really put your mind to it. There are a few good television shows on the subject of money that are extremely helpful to watch, such as *The Suze Orman Show*. And *Money Talk*, heard all over America, is wonderful. Last but not least, you can educate yourself by reading any of the huge number of books available today that will make a difference in your financial future. My favorite author who deals with money is David Bach. His books are fantastic!

It doesn't take a financial genius or a lot of luck to become wealthier or financially secure. All it takes is a small change in the way you look at your discretionary income, and of course in the way you use a small portion of it.

EASIER THAN YOU THINK

32.

DON'T TAKE NOTES

Often when I'm speaking to a group, I'll encourage the audience not to take notes. I do this for two reasons. First of all, it helps people to relax and enjoy the talk instead of focusing on every detail. Second, in my opinion, most of us learn better and have increased insights when we are just listening. Obviously there are times when taking notes is important, but I'm talking about nontechnical information that needs to be absorbed more than memorized.

Many of us have some sort of resistance to not taking notes. For example, when I ask people not to take notes during a presentation, I'll glance down and often notice that a bunch of people in the first few rows are busy taking notes anyway. I suppose some are actually taking notes on the importance of not taking notes!

Many of us attend back-to-school night and frantically take notes about what is being said (I've done this myself). Because we're so busy taking notes, however, we don't really hear what is being said by the instructor. So we miss the entire evening, but boy do we have some great notes to look at.

This theory holds true for classrooms, boardrooms, or offices. We are so anxious to get information down on paper that we more often than not forget the context of our notes. That is, we fail to see the bigger picture of why we are taking notes in the first place. Looking back on our scribbled pages, we are often left to wonder what we were thinking.

Many of us approach life with an intensity that obscures the bigger picture. We grasp at details, holding on tightly, sitting on the edge of our seats. We try so hard with everything we do that we're actually getting in our own way and making life harder than it has to be.

The small change I'm suggesting here is so simple that it's actually difficult for many people: stop trying so hard, listen, and learn. Breathe a little deeper, listen with a quieter mind, and don't worry so much if you don't get every detail just right. You're a lot more competent than you give yourself credit for. You have an inner intelligence that will kick in and take over once you allow that to happen. But your inner intelligence, or wisdom, works only when you are calm and relaxed.

I know this advice runs counter to much of what we are taught in our lives. Usually it's "no pain, no gain," and we end up working harder, faster, and worrying a lot. But when you really look at the truth, you'll see that you're at your best when you are relaxed and calm. Take a look at the most uptight people you know and what do you see? My guess is frustration, stress, anxiety, and an inability to truly solve the daily questions that arise.

I ask people to not take notes. I urge them to relax and let what I have to teach them soak in. A frantic mind with a scribbling pen is a tough barrier for new ideas to surmount. We all have an innate ability to learn, and sometimes we just need to let go a little before we can start the learning process.

See what happens when you stop taking notes, whether at a lecture or at work. You'll be amazed at how receptive your mind is to this new state, and I'll bet you'll be surprised by how much more information you retain.

MY TWO BITS

33.

MY TWO BITS

Over the past ten years or so, I've asked hundreds, possibly even thousands, of people the same question: "If you could, would you change your relationship to the world?" I always phrase it exactly the same way. In all those years the overwhelming majority answer, "Yes, I would."

This nearly unanimous reply has always made me very curious. Since I know that for the most part people don't want to make gigantic changes in their life, the obvious question that remains is this: which small changes are people most willing to make?

Now that we're nearing the end of this book, I suspect that you are deciding which changes you can make that will produce the changes you are looking for while not causing a huge disruption in your life. Maybe the changes will produce more close friendships, a better work opportunity, the lifelong dream of being fit, an improved savings plan, time to read for fun, a solution to a specific problem, or any number of other worthwhile personal goals. Or perhaps your goal is to make a contribution that will make our world a better place for all of us.

Whatever the case may be, I encourage you to keep pondering, even after you finish reading this book, which changes feel right for you. You'll read about several in this section that may spark a great idea for change in your life. Or you may think these suggestions could be helpful for someone else.

Remember, my goal here is not to get everyone thinking and acting in the same ways but instead to focus on those small changes that matter most to you and can produce the largest result. My aim is to encourage you to listen carefully to your own wisdom. That means clearing your mind of all preconceptions and just allowing anything that emerges to enter. My suggestion is to read the stories and suggestions from this chapter and see if they spark an interest or a dormant flame that's been inside of you dying to ignite.

I experienced just such a spark when I heard about Angela. Angela was an eighteen-year-old who was working in an animal shelter as part of a school project. I was so touched by her story that I wrote about it in *Don't Sweat the Small Stuff for Teens.*

The purpose of the shelter was to try to find homes for stray dogs and cats. If no home could be found, the animals were put to sleep. Angela was known for her willingness to work extra hours to find homes for the animals. One day a friend of Angela's came to pick her up at the end of her shift. The two of them were going to a party.

Angela said to her friend, "Before we leave, I have to make one more phone call. There is a woman who expressed an interest in one of our older dogs." That dog's name was Charlie. Her friend, who was annoyed at Angela's persistence and couldn't wait to get out of there, reminded Angela that they were already late. Angela responded calmly, "Be patient. This is something I must do for Charlie."

A few minutes later Angela's friend was glaring at her watch and getting more and more annoyed. Finally, she couldn't stand it anymore and shouted out, "Hurry up already. Forget about it! There are too many animals in here for you to make any difference." At just that moment her friend overheard Angela on the phone saying, "Thank you so much, Mrs. Wright. Sure, I'll meet you down here tomorrow so you can pick up Charlie." As she hung up the phone, she smiled at her friend and said, "Why don't you tell Charlie that I can't make a difference."

That story sure made a difference to me. I was speaking at a book-signing when a teenager in the audience told it, and it made me cry. It reminded me that when I do step forward, all of my actions, regardless of how small they appear to be, make a difference. And since I believe we're all connected to the same spiritual source, I also believe that when one person is kind to someone, it affects everyone in some small way. All of our actions make a difference.

There are so many things we can do. Let's take a look.

34.

GIVE A LITTLE

No doubt you've heard the saying "What goes around comes around." Then there's "Giving is its own reward." And how about "Give and you shall receive"? These sayings and others like them exist for good reason. We all need to be reminded to be more generous.

None of us like to think of ourselves as stingy, but how often have you found an excuse not to help a homeless person on the street, not to give a little more to charity, or not to donate a bit more of your free time to help others? Sure, protecting your time and finances is important. But there's a difference between responsible and being stingy. It's important not to say yes to every request for some of your time or money, but being stingy works against your best interests and against those of everyone else around you.

When Mother Teresa was asked how people could make themselves happier, she often responded, "Go out and serve someone." The truth is that nothing feels better than being generous. Conversely, nothing creates more spiritual emptiness than being stingy.

Obviously, everyone is in a different position when it comes to giving. While one person may be able to make a $10,000 gift with zero financial impact, someone else may be severely burdened by making a ten-dollar gift. Being stingy has nothing to do with the amount you give, but with the attitude and spirit in which you give it.

Being stingy, of course, extends far beyond the financial realm. We can be stingy with our time, our love, our ideas, and our willingness to be of help. We can even be stingy with our willingness to reach out to others or to forgive.

Spiritually, one thing is certain. When we step out of our comfort zone and give a little more than what we are accustomed to giving, be it money, love, time, ideas, forgiveness, or assistance, it comes back to us with interest.

Here's an example of how this small change brings big rewards.

My neighbor John came home from a business trip to India, where hungry children living on the street had reached out to beg for help at every turn. The experience made a big impression on him. John saw for the first time how every little bit makes a difference.

It had always been John's habit when he came home at night to gather his loose change and put it by his wallet, watch, and keys so he could use it the next day for the toll on his commute. But after his trip he started a new habit. He put a large glass jar next to his dresser. He then made a commitment to himself that every day after work, instead of saving the loose change for his own use, he would put it into the jar. Whether he had twenty-five cents or four dollars in change, he'd donate every last cent to the jar. When the jar was full, he rolled the coins, deposited them in the bank, and wrote a check for that amount to support a charity that served children in developing countries.

Just like that, John had found a way to become more generous.

I've talked to hundreds of people, from wealthy CEOs to teenagers who are former gang members, about giving more time and money. And I have never ever met a person who made the decision to do so and then later regretted it. In fact, in every case, a slight increase in generosity brought immense joy and meaning to that person's own life as well as to those he or she was able to help. So why not make the choice to give a little more? Small change goes a long way.

35.

READING IS FOR EVERYONE

Some readers might recognize the following story from my book *Don't Sweat the Small Stuff for Teens*. As you will see, this challenge changed my life. It is one of the most important transformations any of us can make, and I include it here because it is a simple change that positively affects the way we relate to the world.

About twenty-five years ago, my good friend Joseph presented me with an interesting challenge, and now I'm going to present it to you. Like so many people, I believed that I didn't have enough time to read. But Joseph, who was a longtime friend of our family, helped me see that if we're a little bit motivated, all of us have time to read. He knew that one of the reasons people don't read is that they haven't caught the bug. In other words, they don't know how much fun it is to be on the edge of your seat, wondering what's next, unable to put a book down; they haven't yet discovered that reading can completely entertain you wherever you go, any time of the day. Once we're hooked on reading, our lives become so much richer and more interesting.

Had Joseph not posed the following challenge, I might not have read hundreds of the books that I have, and—who knows—I might never have turned out to be a writer.

Here's what he asked me to do. He asked me if I thought I could read eight pages a day, every single day, for a year, from books that were not required reading. (I was eighteen at the time and still in school.) That was it, nothing else, end of contest. At the time I couldn't imagine saying no to a role model of mine. My pride was too great. So I said, sure, I'll read eight pages a day.

Joseph was so dedicated to helping me meet his

challenge that he ensured I got off to a good start by having a box of his favorite books shipped to my front door with a note taped to it. "Richard," it said, "remember our deal: eight pages a day is all it takes."

When I first looked at the assortment of books he had selected, I was a little daunted. Eighteen-year-old that I was at that time, I couldn't resist looking at the number of pages per book and adding them up. As I recall, there were twenty-six books totaling several thousand pages! I almost reneged on my end of the bargain. But then I borrowed a mental trick I had used in sports to prepare myself for the beginning of a game. I repeated the phrase "one step at a time." When you look at any major task in that light, you realize that you don't have to become a champion overnight. That takes years of practice. That first set of books took me a few years to read. Each book expanded my mind in different ways.

That year was a turning point in my life. I had looked at reading as something I had to do, but after agreeing to Joseph's challenge, I started to look at it as something fun to do. Reading took me places I had never been. My imagination grew and my creativity soared. I found myself reading every chance I got. No question about it, I was hooked for life.

Since then, I have upped the ante a bit because I love to read. I have given this challenge to many others, including my two daughters. Here are some numbers to consider. Ten pages a day equals exactly 3,650 pages a year. In ten years, that's 36,500 pages! See how quickly the numbers add up? Of course, if you agree to the challenge, you won't be reading in order to keep score of the number of pages you finish, but rather for the sheer love of it. Reading is one of those remarkable things in life: the more you do it, the more you love it!

Who knows, you might be the reader in your family and not even need any additional incentive to read at all. But maybe someone in your family or someone you care about does need a little push. Why not create a challenge out of it the way Joseph did for me? Or perhaps you can commit to reading ten pages a day to your child or the child of a friend who lives down the street. What a great way to give back to the world. What a gift you would be giving! When you put it into context—ten pages a day—that's really not very much. Most people can read that much during commercial breaks while watching television.

Another idea to expand your mind by reading is a bit more modern and high-tech but fits our times just wonderfully. Recently I was talking to a dear friend on the north coast of California. She had been commuting several hours once a week to a job and was beginning to resent it. One of the things she resented most was that the increased driving time made it difficult for her to find time to read.

Then someone mentioned to her that she could sign up for a books-on-tape service. There was a flat monthly fee, and as soon as she sent one audio book back, the company would immediately send her another through the mail. She said the turnaround time was minimal and the selection was incredible. She told me that this small change literally changed her life.

So whether it's reading ten pages a day in the morning, the evening, or during lunch break or popping an audio book into your car stereo, there are all sorts of ways to enjoy the thrills of reading without taking much time out of your busy schedule.

Reading more is a small change that will fill your mind with immense creative energy and bring un-imaginable fun. Try it today. It's so much easier than you think, and the payoff is huge! In fact, by taking this little challenge, you can become one of the smartest and most well read people around. What have you got to lose?

36.

A LITTLE KINDNESS JUST MIGHT
KEEP THE DOCTOR AWAY

I've always believed that the reason to be kind is that kindness is its own reward. In my opinion, you don't need any other justification whatsoever. However, there are new and exciting studies that claim certain health benefits for acts of kindness. This discovery in combination with what ancient wisdom has to teach us makes for an unbeatable argument.

In recent years a number of scientific studies have concluded that acts of kindness positively affect not only the immune system of the recipient but, almost unbelievably, that of the doer as well! Whether this is true or not remains to be seen, but the suggestion is that when you are kind, you become stronger and healthier. So besides the intrinsic rewards of being kind, we can now add better health as well!

In addition, the Buddhist tradition teaches us that people who are kind and compassionate tend to sleep better and have pleasant dreams, love themselves and are loved by others, and feel peaceful most of the time.

Of course, you'd never want to be kind just to collect some benefit that comes with being kind (that would be unkind, in and of itself); however, knowing about these benefits puts kindness into proper perspective. It shows that kindness is one of our most natural states and a trait we were born to express.

Think about how you feel when you are kind to another person. When was the last time you did something really nice for someone and didn't ask for anything in return? Think of how it made you feel on the inside—relaxed, fulfilled, nourished, and satisfied. How about when someone is kind to you? Don't you feel grateful? Sometimes when I get a beautiful card or letter from someone, or when someone I love does something particularly nice or thoughtful for me, I find that tears come to my eyes. Kindness reminds me of our shared humanity. I even find myself crying when I see someone else being kind to another, whether it's a big deal or not.

Just the other day I was visiting a friend in the hospital. A woman was trying to get in the front door in a wheelchair, but she couldn't quite do it alone. I was going to help her, but a man came running from out of nowhere and beat me to it. He didn't even know her but simply wanted to help. Little things like this inspire me. People love helping each other.

The small change we can all make is to take a few moments each day to remember the power of kindness. You can ask yourself the question: have I been as kind as I could have been today? And if the answer is no, then perhaps you can be a little kinder tomorrow. One thing is certain: if you value the power of kindness and practice it in your daily life, your personal life will be happier, you will experience many terrific benefits, and the world will be a far more peaceful place.

37.

LEAVE THINGS AS YOU FOUND THEM

Suppose you're sitting at your desk paying your bills.
As you finish each one, you toss the used envelope in
the trash. How much more time would it take to set
the recycling bin next to your desk and recycle the
used paper?

The other day I was watering our flowers. When
the phone rang, I ran into the house to answer it. Before
I ran off, I set the hose down on the ground to water
a bush. Thirty minutes later I returned to a flooded
garden and who knows how many wasted gallons of
water.

Again, how much time would it have taken for me

to either turn off the water before answering the phone or, at the very least, walk outside after I had picked up the phone to turn it off? After all, I was on a cordless phone.

When you're at a campground or a public beach, you're often asked to "leave things as you find them." Since I love the ocean, I spend a great deal of time there. Many times over the years I've seen people walk away with shells, starfish, and other sea life whose absence will forever change the environment. I often wonder why people take these specimens. Chances are good that the shells will end up at the bottom of a bag in the back of a garage, or that the starfish will be tossed in the trash when it begins to smell. However, with the smallest amount of discipline each of us could take care to do our part to leave the environment the way we found it.

My cousin Nathan was building a swimming pool. To do so he had to remove a few oak trees, which an arborist had said were sick. The city Nathan lives in and the housing development both agreed to allow him to install his pool and remove the trees provided he replaced the four trees with eight brand-new ones.

That seemed like a reasonable compromise to me, and I'm delighted to report that it seemed fair to him as well. Nathan believes that if you can't leave something exactly the way you found it, you can and should do everything possible to remedy the situation. What I was most impressed with was Nathan's feeling that this regulation applied to him as well as everyone else.

I like to imagine what the world would look like if everyone agreed to leave things as we found them. Or better yet, if everyone agreed to make the world even more beautiful than they found it.

My parents had a rule when my sisters and I were little. They said that if we borrowed someone else's property, we needed to bring it back in better shape than it was in when we borrowed it. If we were staying over at a friend's house, this meant that when we left, it should be cleaner than when we arrived. This rule did two things. First, we were slightly more careful when we were guests because we didn't want to break anything or make any huge messes. We knew that we'd be expected to clean them up. And second, it made us more conscious about our environment. We wanted things to look exactly as they did when we arrived. You don't have to be an extreme environmentalist to want to contribute to a more beautiful world—only someone who loves beauty and cares about other things, be it someone else's property or Mother Nature's beauty.

There are so many little things that you can do that require no more than a small change in the way you look at life. For example, you can stop receiving the newspaper at your house if you already get one at the office. Or if you see trash on the side of the road, you can pick it up the next time you drive or walk by instead of waiting for someone else to do it.

I often shop at the same grocery store, and about a year ago a very nice woman named Diane said that she thought she saw me several days a week at the store. I said, "Yes, I am here a lot." She then asked if I'd be open to a suggestion, and I said that I would be.

It turned out she had a great idea. Diane said, "If you could put the grocery bags in your trunk after you unload your groceries instead of wherever you put them now and simply use them an average of three times instead of once and then recycle them, you'll save a huge number of bags and help our environment each year." She finished by saying, "Richard, I know you're busy, and I wouldn't even ask you to consider this if I thought it would take more than a few extra seconds, but I'm positive that it won't."

Diane's idea was smart. If I use on average four bags each time I shop for groceries, and each bag is double-bagged, that's eight grocery bags I use every time I go shopping. If I use those eight bags three times each instead of just once, I'm probably saving well over one hundred bags a year with absolutely no effort.

There are almost 300 million people in America alone. It's easy to see how quickly the numbers add up, and all we're talking about here are paper grocery bags.

I love this small change because the results are so easy to see and the effort involved is so incredibly minimal. Whenever I leave things as I found them, I feel great about my relationship with the world and know that the world is better off as well. You can't beat that.

38.

MAKE A SMALL DIFFERENCE IN
SOMEONE'S LIFE
EVERY DAY

Several years ago I gave a lecture to a room full of enthusiastic people in a large U.S. city. I felt that I had done a good job and covered a variety of topics. Almost immediately upon returning home, I started receiving dozens of letters, e-mails, and phone calls. One hundred percent of this response was caused by a single suggestion. It also happened to be the simplest suggestion I made, the one that required the smallest change.

That suggestion was to try every single day to make a small difference in someone else's life.

Rather than give you my own list of ways to make a difference, I'll share with you a few of the ideas that came directly from that audience. Each suggestion might take anywhere from a minimum of five seconds of your time to a maximum of five minutes. All are very simple, and only a few of them cost anything. Even with those that do, the cost is nominal.

The personal benefit, however, is huge in terms of how you'll feel when you go to bed at night. As you think back on your day, you'll realize that you made a positive difference in the life of another human being. Sometimes the people you help will know it was you who did it, and other times they will never know. Sometimes your efforts are noticed and appreciated; other times they are not. None of this matters. All that matters is that you know and that you get the positive feelings that result.

One person from that event even told me that she and some friends were going to meet every other month to discuss additional ways to be of service to others so that their ideas would always remain fresh.

Almost everyone who practices this strategy tells me it's one of their favorite parts of the day. With almost zero effort, they get to feel good, they know they are making a positive difference, and they never again complain that one person can't make a difference. They now know that each of us does make a difference every single day simply by the way we act in the world. Plus, we get to imagine a world where everyone else is doing the same thing. When we try to make a difference, even on a very small scale, it's extremely satisfying and nourishing.

Here are ideas for ways you can brighten the day of other people. Notice that in every case the change to your own routine is extremely minimal.

- Pick up litter in someone else's yard or property.
- Pay someone else's toll behind you on the bridge or expressway.
- Smile at a cashier and tell them what a great job they are doing.
- Send a "Thinking of You" greeting card in the mail, the old-fashioned way.
- Do the same with e-mail.

EASIER THAN YOU THINK

- Call someone just to say, "I love you," or for some other nice reason. Have no agenda and don't ask anything of the person you call.
- Think of people in your life who do many things for others. Realize that they are probably not used to being thanked very often. So call just to say thank you on behalf of all they do. Again, don't ask for anything in return.
- When you're in a conversation and someone wants to be right, let them. You'll be surprised at the difference this makes. And what do you care anyway? Your goal is to make that person happy!
- Send an anonymous donation to your favorite charity (even to two) and don't tell anyone about it. There is something very intrinsically rewarding about giving money without tooting your own horn.
- On a similar note, if a friend is in need, consider doing something to help but don't ever let him or her know you did it.
- Smile at strangers on the street until you get someone to smile back. Eventually someone will.

- This came from an eleven-year-old girl: clean up your sister's room. Pretty nice sister, don't you think? You could do the same for any one of your family members or friends, or you could do the dishes even when it's not your turn, or clean out the garage without being asked, and so forth.
- Cut someone else's grass. A gentleman who shared a property line with his neighbor was mowing his own grass and appeared to be mowing his neighbor's as well. So I asked him. He said, "Oh sure, I'm out here anyway. Why not save my neighbor the trouble?" Imagine if everyone thought like him?
- Pick some flowers and bring them home for your loved one.

I could go on and on. But more important, you can create your own list of ideas and start incorporating them into your life. Making others feel good and doing nice things for people simply makes you feel better in the process—a win-win situation. This small change is well worth the effort.

39.

SAIL AWAY WITH SMALL CHANGE

In the introduction to this book, I mentioned my love of watching sailboats darting across the open water. I also discussed how the slightest shift in the rudder or wheel in the wrong direction can put the boat many miles off course. Yet the reverse is also true: with a tiny shift back in the right direction, the boat is back on course. All it takes is a slight adjustment.

That's the nature of small change. A little effort goes a long way. My hope in writing this book was not only to share with you some specific ideas that can improve the quality of your life, but just as important, to get you thinking about how easy it is to make small changes in your life. I hope you've seen just how powerful the results can be when you do make positive small changes in your life. A few carefully selected small changes can make life easier and more enjoyable every single day.

In "A Penny for Your Thoughts," we discussed how one tiny shift in your attitude can make the difference between misery and happiness. In "Take Five," you saw that making a small step back instead of overreacting or reacting simply out of fear can radically reduce your stress and make your life so much better day to day. In "Turning on a Dime," you learned small changes that will enable you to adapt and respond appropriately to many of life's twists and turns. And last, in "My Two Bits," we talked about the small changes you can make that affect the world you live in and in turn make you feel better about yourself. The book has gone from the inside out and back again, and I hope it has shown you the power of small change.

So many of the changes we're talking about are not only small but tiny, and so simple to put into practice. For example, we've seen that saving a few dollars a day can really add up. We've also seen that putting "first things first" can help us become more successful at work. We've seen dozens of other examples where a slight change of heart, an awareness of something amiss in our thinking, or a shift in our behavior can make all the difference.

I hope that this book has helped you see that you have the capacity and the power to make whatever small changes you want in your own life. It's absolutely up to you. Whether it's emotional, physical, behavioral, spiritual, intrapersonal, or you name it, all you have to do is imagine that you're on that sailboat and you're the one making the adjustment. Small change never requires a huge effort. Instead, it's a minimal adjustment that fits right into your life.

Now that you're moving in the right direction, you'll be sailing in open water, relaxed, and with the wind blowing through your hair. My guess is that you'll soon arrive at your ideal destination . . . right on course!

ACKNOWLEDGMENTS

It might seem that writing a book is a one-person job when in fact there are many people involved who deserve a great deal of credit. I wish to express my deepest gratitude to all who supported and assisted me in writing this book.

First to Linda Chester, my literary agent, who demonstrated time and again that patience and excellence are virtues to be admired. Thank you for pushing me to go the extra mile and for being my partner and friend in what I believe to be an important and valuable book. And to Gary Jaffe for all the help you have provided me during this time. Your resourcefulness and sense of humor are much appreciated.

To Steve Hanselman for inviting me to be a part of the Harper San Francisco family and for your keen insights into the very heart of this book—from the initial concept to the title, thank you. To Kyra Ryan for your immensely valuable editorial contributions and insights, as well as the friendship we developed along the way. You were brilliant.

To Marvin Levin for spending many unselfish hours with me sharing your ideas, insights, stories, and wisdom. This book would not have been the same without your help. Thank you for being so accessible to me and for being my lifelong friend.

To Gideon Weil for your magical editorial skills; you have an amazing way with words. Even when you cut out an entire paragraph from a chapter, you found a way to make me feel good about it! You are amazing. To Mark Tauber at Harper San Francisco for your wonderful ideas on how to share this book with the public; and to everyone at Harper who has worked so hard to make this book all it can be. I appreciate all of you very much. To Linda Michaels, my foreign agent and close friend, thank you for sharing this book with people all over the world!

To Ken Bradford, thank you for your perspective and keen insights and for helping me obtain a level of quiet that I had not been able to achieve on my own. You are a shining light in my life. To Benjamin Shield, my best friend in the world, who encourages me through good times and bad and who helps me make many "small changes" in my life. Thank you for being you.

To my assistant and good friend Susan Miller, thank you for making it possible for me to indulge in my need to become a bit isolated when I write. And finally thank you to the loves of my life—Kris, Jazzy, and Kenna. The three of you make my life complete and I thank you for supporting me while I immerse myself in what I love so much.

THE *Easier Than You Think* TO DO LIST

A Penny for Your Thoughts

_____

_____

_____

_____

_____

_____

_____

_____

_____

Take Five

_____

_____

_____

_____

_____

_____

_____

_____

The Easier Than You Think *To Do List*

Turning on a Dime

_____

_____

_____

_____

_____

_____

_____

_____

_____

My Two Bits

_____

_____

_____

_____

_____

_____

_____

_____

_____